FERTILITY

Why Microbes, Weight & Nutrition Matter

Clare Fleishman MS RDN

Clare Fleishman MS RDN
Origin Story Press

Printed in the United States of America
First Printing 2022
First Edition 2022

ISBN: 979-8-218-02402-4

10 9 8 7 6 5 4 3 2 1

To my parents, Marcella and Herbert Aigner

Thank you for my brothers and sisters: Michael, Mary, Kathleen, Joan, Andrew, Stephen, and John.

Life is rich.

"Go confidently in the direction of your dreams."

– Henry David Thoreau

DISCLAIMER

The information provided in this book should not be used to diagnose or treat any medical condition. For diagnosis or treatment of any medical problem, consult your physician. The publisher and author are not responsible for any specific health or allergy needs that may require medical supervision and are not liable for any damages or negative consequences from any treatment, action, application, or preparation, to any person reading or following the information in this book. References are provided for informational purposes only and do not constitute an endorsement of any websites or other sources. Although the author and publisher have made every effort to ensure that the information in this book was correct at press time, the author and publisher do not assume and hereby disclaim any liability to any party for any loss, damage, or disruption caused by errors or omissions, whether such errors or omissions result from negligence, accident, or any other cause.

TABLE OF CONTENTS

INTRODUCTION

You have decided. You want to have a baby.

The choice may not have been easy. Bringing a child into a world struggling with a lingering pandemic, political unrest, and climate change is viewed by some as irresponsible or uncaring. Add to that exorbitant student debt, unaffordable childcare and rising housing prices and many young people may delay the decision to start a family.[1]

If all that doesn't sound too ominous, know this: the payoff is unsurpassed. Creating a new life or two, or more can bring unconditional love to your time on earth.

But if it turns out to be a struggle to conceive, it may come as a surprise, especially after so many years of trying to avoid unwanted pregnancy. Still, our bodies were born for this; passing DNA to the next generation has been the glorious and consummate plan for human beings since time began. Procreation is the driving force behind evolution. That's why sex feels good and babies are so adorable. But for some, it is a struggle to conceive. Modern life with all its pollution, stress, junk food, and workplace demands is not always biologically conducive to creating new life. Our bodies push back, making infertility, miscarriages and problem pregnancies more likely. Nonetheless, identifying the source of such obstacles to healthy reproduction can point the way to better lifestyle choices.

Wherever you are in the quest to have a child, prepare like a life depended on it. It does. Get ready by learning the newest information about enhancing fertility. Then make an action plan. This book explores the latest research on how microbes, weight, and nutrition are fundamental to fertility and reproductive health. Other publications on fertility may address these areas separately or just briefly along with other influences such as pollution and chemicals. This review, however, is intended as a comprehensive record of the available literature on microbes, weight, and nutrition and how each impacts fertility in both women and men. It leans heavily on evidence-based research. Inspirational stories or anecdotal evidence are largely absent because one person's experience doesn't prove much of anything (though it may spark a hypothesis). Also avoided are personal blogs and wellness websites, which may obscure the facts behind opinion, or worse, alongside commercial advertisements.

Instead, many hundreds of studies from peer-reviewed journals and other respected sources were scoured to arrive at the closest possible truths.

This format makes it an easy and reliable resource for healthcare practitioners who work in obstetrics and gynecology as well as in fertility clinics. Doctors, nurses, nurse practitioners and dietitians who work in these areas will find the compiled information useful in their practices, with the assurance that it is based only on trustworthy sources. But no one requires a PhD in microbiology to understand the content.

When possible, simpler language is used rather than the dense semantics of academia. In addition, a helpful glossary explains the various vocabulary involved in reproduction as well as terms not used in daily conversation.

As a complete work, the information and extensive data can lead to an action plan for enhancing fertility and reproductive health.

Part One: Fertility, the Essence

Fertility begins after puberty, in the early teenage years for both women and men.[2]

For women, fertility declines due to normal, age-related changes that occur in the ovaries. A woman's best reproductive years are in her 20s. Fertility gradually declines in the 30s, particularly after age 35.

- *30 years of age*: 20 out of 100 fertile women trying to get pregnant in 1 cycle will be successful.
- *40 years of age*: fewer than 5 out of 100 will be fruitful.

Men continue to produce sperm throughout their lives, though quality may suffer in later years.

More people need help with fertility these days. One data set from the Centers for Disease Control and Prevention (CDC) suggests that more than 10% of American women seek fertility treatment over their lifetimes.[3] For a variety of reasons, many women are waiting longer to have children. Beyond college and a healthy stretch of time after career launch and then finding a mate, a woman finds herself in her 30s, right around the time fertility starts declining. It may come as a revelation to young couples, but birth control only became available about the same time their parents were young. For the first time in history, one could choose (though not 100% foolproof) when to have children, or not. Of course, abstinence was always an option but not very effective. These days, considering the major life changes and financial commitments that parenting entails, many young couples choose to wait.

On the outside, a woman may still look young, but her eggs are aging: both the quality and quantity of her eggs decline gradually. Fertility drops.

Some modern couples may believe that freezing young eggs or using assisted reproductive technology (ART) procedures such as in vitro fertilization (IVF) are workarounds for busy millennials. Planned parenthood can also mean getting pregnant on demand, right? Not really. "Birth control" has always been an imperfect science. In fact, long-written biological imperatives favor parents who are limber enough to nurture a child through to adulthood. Overriding the *force majeure* of evolution is not easy, thus success rates of assisted treatments are also impacted by age and other factors.

Taking steps to evaluate infertility is suggested when a couple fails to achieve pregnancy after 12 months of regular, unprotected sexual intercourse. As many as 48 million couples and 186 million individuals worldwide experience difficulty becoming pregnant.[4] But make no assumptions based on the heavy lifting done by the woman in pregnancy. A man can be the source of infertility too. Sometimes the cause is not found.[5]

Causes of infertility are many, not just age.[6] Anatomical or genetic anomalies, systemic or neurological diseases, infections, trauma, and antibody development can all be implicated.

In the female, infertility may be caused by a range of abnormalities of the ovaries, uterus, fallopian tubes, and the endocrine system.

In males, the most common causes are problems in the ejection of semen, absence or low levels of sperm, or abnormal shape (morphology) and movement (motility) of the sperm.

Environmental toxins[7] and an unhealthy lifestyle[8] may contribute. Exercise-induced amenorrhea (absence of menstruation) and being underweight are two lifestyle conditions that may cause infertility. And as obesity rates soar, sperm quality has inextricably dropped. In addition, scientists are exploring the causes of infertility in some novel new areas.[9]

Part Two: Female Fertility and the Microbiome

The Female Reproductive System

A woman's vagina teems with live microbes. They are as unique to her as the color of her skin or hair. But they are far more important though.

These microbes support the foundations underpinning many facets of reproductive health. They, in a sense, represent the future. Unfortunately, not much attention is paid until they cause trouble such as itching or oozing. Scientists have found that certain mixes of microbes are linked with problems like vaginosis and sexually transmitted diseases. Pathogens are more likely to spread when specific microbes are present or absent.

FYI: *The microbiome refers to the collective genomes of bacteria, viruses, bacteriophages, protozoa, and fungi that symbiotically inhabit the human body.*[10] *These microbial cells outnumber human cells by an estimated tenfold. The Human Microbiome Project,*[11] *a summation of multiple projects undertaken across the globe, seeks to design strategies to manipulate microbiota to optimize its performance.*

The female reproductive system is home to vast numbers of microorganisms. The Human Microbiome Project found that vaginal microbiota accounts for nearly 10% of the whole human sum of microbiota. But in the last few years, mounting evidence has also shown the presence of microorganisms (though 10,000 times less concentration than in the vagina) in the upper female reproductive system, which includes the ovaries, Fallopian tubes, and uterus. Until recently, this upper region was thought to be sterile.[12] An excellent figure available online summarizes the different bacteria reported thus far in the different areas of the female reproductive system.[13]

Lactobacillus is the most abundant genus throughout the female reproductive system. These resident microbes markedly contribute to health. Alterations have been linked to several gynecological diseases including chronic endometritis, endometriosis, pelvic inflammatory disease, and gynecological cancers.[14]

NOTE: New taxonomy changes have reclassified some lactobacilli as will be seen in the most current literature. The microbe remains the same. Bifidobacteria have not changed, but nomenclature changes are expected soon.

For an example, see this 2021 study[15] online where *Lactobacillus salivarius* is now named or classified as *Ligilactobacillus salivarius*. As most research cited here was reported before these changes, the original names will be retained.

Old Name	**New Name**
Lactobacillus casei	*Lacticaseibacillus casei*
Lactobacillus paracasei	*Lacticaseibacillus paracasei*
Lactobacillus rhamnosus	*Lacticaseibacillus rhamnosus*
Lactobacillus plantarum	*Lactiplantibacillus plantarum*
Lactobacillus brevis	*Levilactobacillus brevis*
Lactobacillus salivarius	*Ligilactobacillus salivarius*
Lactobacillus fermentum	*Limosilactobacillus fermentum*
Lactobacillus reuteri	*Limosilactobacillus reuteri*

One recent review[16] describes the many efforts made to try to establish the composition and role of a "healthy" female reproductive system microbiome as well as the effects of a disrupted microbiota on human reproduction and fertility. Again, the female reproductive system microbiota is vital for women's health and fetal development. Disturbingly, negative effects can carry over to the next generation, in the predisposition to diseases that may develop later in life, into adulthood.[17]

Upper Reproductive System

Continuity in microbial communities exists at six sites along the female reproductive tract.[18] However, a lower count of bacteria is found in the ovaries, the Fallopian tubes, and the uterus for these possible reasons:

- The cervical barrier may hamper the ascension of microbes from the vagina.
- Immune reactions may occur.
- Environmental factors may prompt the growth of specific taxa (units of biological classification, from kingdom to subspecies).

Nevertheless, the microbiota may be able to modulate the functions of both endometrial cells and the local immune system as well as prevent uterine infections by both competing with pathogenic microorganisms and producing protective molecules.[19] Moreover, it appears that similar microbiome profiles are found in the upper system as in the vagina.[20]

Lower Reproductive System

In healthy, reproductive-age women, the vaginal microbiome accounts for about 1 billion bacteria per gram of vaginal fluid. Unlike healthy microbiota in other regions such as the gastrointestinal tract, vaginal microbiota is distinctive for its low diversity. Lactobacilli account for up to 95% of total bacteria.[21]

A healthy vaginal microbiota is simple compared to the diversity found elsewhere in the body. Yet it is dynamic, changing throughout the life of a female.

Composition changes over a women's life:[22]

- **Childhood**: *Escherichia coli* and anaerobes predominate.
- **Puberty**: Estrogen rises; this leads to glycogen production, which is essential for lactobacilli growth and colonization. The dominance of lactobacilli is sustained during the reproductive years.
- **Post-menopausal**: Estrogen decreases, leading to a higher pH—less acidic—and lactobacilli numbers fall. Pathogens move in and colonize, making a profile similar to that in bacterial vaginosis.

"A balanced environment of vaginal microbiota acts as a gatekeeper of female reproductive system and plays a key role in protecting it from infections that may ascend to upper reproductive tract and lead to many gynecological complications," wrote the authors of a recent review, titled "Probiotics and the envisaged role in treating human infertility."[23]

Which *Lactobacillus* Species Are Dominant?

The vaginal microbiota in healthy reproductive-age women is mainly composed of one or a few *Lactobacillus* species, which represent more than 90% of the total microbiota.[24]

Lactobacillus crispatus, Lactobacillus gasseri, Lactobacillus iners, and *Lactobacillus jensenii* are the most represented in the vagina of healthy women. It's not clear why other species such as *Lactobacillus helveticus* or *Lactobacillus acidophilus* are not present.[25]

The presence of *Lactobacillus* spp. has been considered a substantial biomarker for the assessment of healthy vaginal microbiota. Yet despite the dominance of just a few species, further exploration found marked differences in healthy women (asymptomatic for disease).

Jacque Ravel and colleagues conducted intriguing research with 396 asymptomatic North American women who represented four ethnic groups (White, Black, Hispanic, and Asian). After sampling, species composition was identified by barcoded 16S rRNA genes. The study titled "Vaginal microbiome of reproductive-age women" appeared in *Proceedings of National Academy of Sciences USA.*[26]

This groundbreaking research revealed five distinct "community state types (CSTs)" depending on the abundance of the bacteria identified. CST-I, -II, -III, and -V are dominated by *Lactobacillus crispatus, Lactobacillus gasseri, Lactobacillus iners*, and *Lactobacillus jensenii*, respectively. These four main groups were isolated primarily from White and Asian women.

The researchers found dominant bacteria to be different in the sample groups:

- Grade I is dominated by *Lactobacillus crispatus (in 26% of sample)*
- Grade II: *Lactobacillus gasseri* (6%)
- Grade III: *Lactobacillus iners* (34%)
- Grade V: *Lactobacillus jensenii* (5%)

But what happened to Grade IV?

Puzzlingly, Grade IV was not dominated by *Lactobacillus.* Instead, organisms far more diverse including *Gardnerella, Prevotella, Corynebacterium, Atopobium, Megasphaera* and *Sneathia* were present. Adding to the disparity (and perhaps troublesome), sexual activity and the transition through CST-IV are risk factors for bacterial vaginosis (BV).[27]

Again, Ravel's community state types (CSTs) depend on the abundance of the bacteria identified. Increasingly, it is clear that what is "normal" or a healthy vaginal microbiome may be different for different communities.

Different Women, Different Microbes

No core vaginal microbiota exists for all women.

Analysis of vaginal microbiota of White, Black, Hispanic and Asian women reveals big differences. The CST-IV profile—not dominated by *Lactobacillus*—is also common in asymptomatic women (no bacterial vaginosis) depending on their racial background. This CST-IV profile was found mainly in Black and Hispanic women.

The percentage of women with a lower genital tract dominated by *Lactobacillus:*

- 90% White
- 80% Asian
- 60% Hispanic
- 37% to 60% Black

The difference in microbiota profiles in these populations may reflect not only racial or genetic predisposition to one or other types of bacteria, but also geographic, social, and/or economic factors.

This distinction is striking, and important. Microbial composition with higher diversity and less lactobacilli dominance appears to be closely associated with genital inflammation, as measured by cervicovaginal pro-inflammatory cytokines and the presence of activated immune cells.[28]

Unfortunately, such inflammation is associated with a number of adverse reproductive outcomes, including increased incidence of sexually transmitted infections (STIs) and poor obstetric events. Thus such a microbial community may not be optimal. Yet the possibility exists that genital inflammation may be an advantage in specific contexts, contributing to the high prevalence of diverse microbiota in certain populations.[29]

Lactobacilli and Vaginal Health

Lactobacilli and related organisms appear to help maintain vaginal health by several mechanisms:

Lactic Acid Production

The process begins when the hormone estrogen triggers an accumulation of glycogen in vaginal epithelial cells (the protective inner lining of the vagina). This leads lactobacilli to produce lactic acid. Lactic acid is the star performer in a normal or healthy vaginal milieu. As the name states, it's an acid, so if you can recall from high school chemistry class, pH drops down below 4.5.

A low pH (acidic) is anathema to pathogens. The bad actors that induce vaginosis shrivel up and die. Researchers believe that this acidic environment is also inhospitable to the scourge called human immunodeficiency virus (HIV) as well as sexually transmitted diseases—no picnic either– including gonorrhea, Chlamydia and herpes simplex.[30]

Hydrogen Peroxide and Bacteriocins Production

Some species of lactobacilli also produce hydrogen peroxide and/or bacteriocins, which may contribute to the suppression of other bacterial species. Hydrogen peroxide has also been shown to harm vaginal pathogens and may increase pathogen sensitivity to antibiotics.[31]

Physical Barrier

Adhesion by the lactobacilli to epithelial cells creates a physical barrier against pathogens' adhesion. Lactobacilli do this by displacement and competition for nutrients via multiple mechanisms.[32]

Immune Activation

The immune modulatory effects of vaginal microbiota can prevent or promote susceptibility to infection by reproductive tract pathogens. Lactobacilli may in part mediate the effects through the production of organic acid metabolites including lactic acid as well as acetate, propionate, butyrate, and succinate.[33]

As noted before, the makeup of lactobacilli in the lower female reproductive system is related to racial, genetic, geographic, and social factors. But the vaginal microbiota is also influenced by environmental factors, such as hygiene habits, sexual exposure, change of sexual partners, and use and type of contraceptives, all of which may be responsible for microbial fluctuations over time.[34] The significance of these variations is being explored.

An excellent diagram (available online) depicts the factors influencing the structure and composition of the cervicovaginal microbiota.[35]

We can see from the evidence that the vaginal microbiota plays a vital role in maintaining a healthy environment free of pathogens. The sophisticated and complex interplay is crucial to protecting the female reproductive system as it prepares for pregnancy and healthy children.

Now we will consider common maladies, which may interfere with this optimization of the female reproductive system.

Dysbiosis in Female Reproductive Diseases

***Dysbiosis**: an imbalance in the microbial community due to the gain or loss of microbes or changes in their relative abundance and associated with disease.*

Bacterial Vaginosis

Bacterial vaginosis is the most common vaginal disorder for women of reproductive age, affecting 23–29% of women globally.[36]

Traditional treatment consists of antibiotics, including metronidazole or clindamycin, but about half of women treated have a recurrence within one-year post-treatment.[37]

Boric acid is another therapy that has shown some success, thought to be through the inhibition of biofilm formation, which may decrease host inflammation in the mucosal site, promoting epithelial repair.[38]

Bacterial vaginosis is characterized by an interruption of commensal bacterial habitat in the vagina and colonization by pathogenic microorganisms.[39] Adverse changes include increased pro-inflammatory cytokines, altered immunity and epithelial barrier disruption.[40]

Lactobacillus spp. drop markedly as pathogenic bacteria (*Gardnerella* spp., *Atopobium* spp., *Prevotella* spp., and *Mobiluncus* spp.) colonize.[41]

Several events ensue:

As lactobacilli decrease, lactic acid levels also fall leading to a higher pH.[42] Then the hostile pathogens grow bolder, inducing the production of enzymes that disrupt the mucus coating vaginal epithelium.[43] This coating is a strong barrier against infection. Pathogens can then wield another weapon by forming a biofilm that allows other pathogenic species to adhere.[44]

Lactobacilli species are the workhorses in the vagina.

In addition to maintaining vaginal health, lactobacilli may have different biological activities that contribute to fertility and healthy pregnancy:[45]

- Inhibition of colonization and growth of harmful microbes that can compromise fertility
- Enhanced implantation of the embryo through angiogenesis (growth of new blood vessels)

- Induced immunomodulation (modification of the immune response) activities involved in implantation and tolerance of embryo and fetus

When bacterial vaginosis takes hold, the resulting dysbiosis can lead to infertility. BV may factor in nearly 20% of women suffering from infertility.[46] BV is linked to higher rates of intra-amniotic infection, premature delivery, spontaneous abortion, and infertility.[47]

BV may be implicated in infertility through a variety of mechanisms including immune activation, inflammation, and toxin production.[48]

Bacterial vaginosis also figures in endometriosis, pelvic inflammatory disease, and tubal blockage as well as elevating the risk of sexually transmitted diseases.[49]

Specific probiotics have been successful in preventing recurrent bacterial vaginosis.[50]

Endometriosis

Chronic endometritis is a persistent inflammation of the mucus membrane lining the uterus. It is mainly caused by infection with common bacteria such as *Enterobacteria, Streptococcus* species, and *Enterococcus faecalis*, as well as *Chlamydia, Mycoplasma,* and *Ureaplasma* species, along with a decreased abundance of beneficial lactobacilli bacteria.[51] Chronic endometritis is found in up to 40% of infertile patients. An abnormal endometrial microbiota has been associated with implantation failure, pregnancy loss, and other gynecological and obstetrical conditions.[52] Indeed, reduced colonization of lactobacilli in the endometrium also led to poor reproductive outcomes in other studies.[53]

A 2022 review concluded that even though there is no consensus on the endometrial bacterial core, a healthy endometrial microbiota should be considered a group of microorganisms that is permissive for embryo implantation and live birth, regardless of the minimum presence of pathogenic bacteria.[54]

Moreover, in the transfer of embryos in IVF procedures, endometrial dysbiosis and its implications in the transfer catheter bacterial cultures are linked to IVF failure.[55]

Unfortunately, because endometriosis is often asymptomatic, it is rarely suspected, diagnosed, and treated.

Pelvic Inflammatory Disease (PID)

Pelvic inflammatory disease (PID), as its name suggests, is an inflammation of the upper genital tract. It is caused by infection with *Escherichia coli*, additional BV-associated pathogens (*Atopobium vaginae, Sneathia sanguinegens*, and *Sneathia amnionii*, among others) or sexually transmitted bacteria (*Chlamydia trachomatis, Mycoplasma genitalium*, and *Neisseria gonorrhoeae*).[56] In addition to causing abdominal pain, PID affects the uterus and fallopian tubes, potentially leading to infertility.

Polycystic Ovary Syndrome (PCOS)

Polycystic Ovary Syndrome (PCOS) is a common endocrine disorder, characterized by inflammation and excess secretion of testosterone. The majority of women with PCOS have ovarian dysfunction, irregular bleeding, acne, hirsutism (male-like hair growth), and infertility.[57]

All of these conditions—BV, PCOS, PID, and endometriosis—are in deep with the microbial disarray that can lead to infertility.

The Microbiome in Infertility Treatments

Female infertility is rising. It can be caused by numerous factors: hormonal changes, tubal changes, uterine pathologies, maternal age, and systemic or genetic diseases.[58] Though much has been learned about the causes of infertility, rates of successful pregnancies with available therapies such as embryo transfer through in vitro fertilization (IVF) remain low.[59]

Ovulation disorders are blamed for the largest proportion of female infertility. As a woman ages, Dr. Shanna Swan PhD reports in her 2021 book Count Down,[60] her number of eggs declines precipitously. From 300,000 eggs at puberty, a woman may have about 25,000 at age 37 and 1000 at menopause.

In addition, a fertility center report illustrated how miscarriage and chromosomal abnormalities increase dramatically with age. The miscarriage rate from age 25 to 35 years is 10% and rises to 40% at age 40 and 60% at age 50. Down syndrome risk rises from 1/900 pregnancies from age 25 to 35 years and 1/100 at age 40 and 1/10 at age 50.[61]

The good news? The microbiome presents a new frontier in attempts to improve those rates.

Why?

First, infertile women host a different microbiota than healthy and fertile women, as concluded in a recent review of the evidence.[62]

For example, one pilot study found that infertile women—when compared to women with a history of fertility—more often had *Ureaplasma* in the vagina and *Gardnerella* in the cervix.[63]

In another analysis, specific bacteria were identified that distinguished the idiopathic (cause unknown) infertile women from other groups.[64]

Assisted Reproductive Technology (ART)

Support for infertile couples to achieve successful pregnancies is generally considered under the umbrella term of assisted reproductive technology (ART). In ART, the cycle begins with ovarian stimulation, egg retrieval and in vitro fertilization of eggs. One or more embryos are then transferred into the uterine cavity, usually by passing a catheter through the cervical os (opening).

As stated before, many transfers do not result in a pregnancy. A lot of factors affect success. One new focus of research is how our microbes figure in ART success.

Microbiota in healthy women of procreative age have lactobacilli dominance and low diversity in the reproductive organs. (Interestingly, high diversity is usually seen as a positive in most other areas such as the gut and oral cavity.)

A different microbiota profile such as one with fewer lactobacilli and higher diversity is considered dysbiosis. Researchers questioned if dysbiosis was a factor in IVF success rates.

Indeed, dysbiosis appears to be a significant factor.

Deviations from the low-diversity vaginal microbiome have been significantly correlated with decreased pregnancy rates after IVF.[65]

The microbial composition of the reproductive tract is strongly correlated to successful IVF cycles.

In one study, the beneficial role of specific lactobacilli species in improving fertility was quite evident. A 40% pregnancy rate was observed after IVF cycles in 84 patients with *Lactobacillus*-dominated vaginal microbiota. But of those women with bacterial vaginosis (*Gardnerella vaginalis* and/or *Atopobium vaginae*), only 9% were able to conceive.[66]

As noted before, the endometrial microbial population also must be considered in infertility. Infectious bacteria may dominate in an often-undetected disorder.

In a 2018 study, researchers in Japan evaluated endometrial fluid of 79 IVF patients and its impact on reproductive outcomes. Results showed stark differences. Only 38% of infertile women undergoing IVF presented with a *Lactobacillus*-dominated microbiota in the endometrium. Healthy volunteers presented with 86%. Moreover, patients achieving pregnancy after IVF had an average lactobacilli content of 96.5% suggesting that a *Lactobacillus*-dominated endometrium might favor implantation.[67]

In addition, the replacement of a community dominated by *Lactobacillus* with pathogenic bacteria may be associated with implantation failure or early spontaneous abortion in patients undergoing assisted reproductive technology (ART) treatment.[68]

And in another study, the presence of a non-*Lactobacillus*-dominated microbiota in a receptive endometrium was associated with significant decreases in implantation, pregnancy, ongoing pregnancy, and live birth rates.[69]

However, this link is not always supported.[70]

IVF Transfer

The transfer of embryo(s) into the uterine cavity by passing a catheter through the cervical opening is a delicate procedure. Microbes take part in a successful transfer. Several studies support the hypothesis that the reproductive-tract microbiome on the day of embryo transfer affects pregnancy outcome.

According to one study, colonizing the transfer-catheter tip with *Lactobacillus crispatus* at the time of embryo transfer may increase the rates of implantation and live birth rate while decreasing the rate of infection. Conversely, isolation of pathogens such as *Enterococci, Enterobacteriaceae, Streptococci, Staphylococci*, and/or Gram-negative bacteria is correlated with lower implantation rate, decreased number of at-term pregnancies and an increased number of miscarriages. [71]

In a study of 110 women at the time of embryo transfer, the clinical pregnancy rates were 57.1% in the group of patients without growth and 29.6% in the group with positive microbial growth from catheter tips.[72]

Importantly, only specific lactobacilli species are dominant in the healthy flora; these species are likely to play a pivotal role in maintaining a supportive environment for implantation and future pregnancy outcome.

It's encouraging news. The microbiome may prove to be a worthy target to improve IVF outcomes. Researchers believe that reducing the numbers of bacterial pathogens in the reproductive tract and increasing the proportion of beneficial *Lactobacillus* could improve reproductive outcomes.[73]

How to do this? Two lines of attack: Antibiotics and/or probiotics.

Boosting Fertility by Altering the Microbiome

Antibiotics

Antibiotics are the go-to treatment for infections in the reproductive tract.

In one study, antibiotic therapy resulted in chronic endometritis resolution in 82% of patients; the disease persisted in the remaining women. Chronic endometritis (CE) is rampant—estimated at up to 40%—in women with unexplained infertility. Women with cured chronic endometritis showed a higher pregnancy rate and live birth rate in comparison with both women with persistent disease and women without a chronic endometritis diagnosis.[74]

Endometriosis is also frequently observed in recurrent miscarriages (defined as three or more miscarriages before 20 weeks of pregnancy). Antibiotic therapy improved the outcomes significantly in a recent study.[75]

A 2018 review included a total of 796 patients from five studies. Antibiotic therapy for CE improved implantation, clinical pregnancy, ongoing pregnancy, and live birth rate after CE was resolved in a subsequent IVF cycle.[76]

Antibiotics are quite effective in killing off harmful bacteria. However, their scorched earth modus operandi is being increasingly questioned. Antibiotics can wipe out beneficial organisms, which are critical in reaching healthy fertility. Beneficial microbes struggling to hold on to their turf are decimated, collateral damage that may not have to be tolerated.

There may be a better way: probiotics.

PROBIOTICS

Another strategy to modify the reproductive tract microbiome is to use probiotics. By definition, probiotics are 'live microorganisms that, when administered in adequate amounts, confer a health benefit on the host.'[77]

Because of their dominance in a healthy reproductive tract, *Lactobacillus* strains, in particular, are being studied for usage in populating the tract and displacing pathogens. Specific probiotics may promote *Lactobacillus* stability, increasing the presence of immunomodulatory products such as hydrogen peroxide and lactic acid, as well as decreasing inflammation.

Female fertility may be improved with probiotics by safeguarding a lactobacilli-rich reproductive microbiome to prevent infections, which can lead to bacterial vaginosis, preterm birth and infertility.[78]

Because bacterial vaginosis (BV) is a dysbiotic condition that can lead to poor reproductive outcomes, researchers designed trials to find out if probiotics could help.

In an early study, 40 Nigerian women with BV were given capsules containing strains of *Lactobacillus rhamnosus* and *Lactobacillus reuteri* or metronidazole gel (an antibiotic). A 90% recovery rate ensued in the probiotic group with a significantly lower recovery seen in the antibiotic group.[79]

A few years later, in a study of 39 women with BV, a randomly selected test group received vaginal tablets containing several *Lactobacillus* strains (*L. brevis, L. salivarius, and L. plantarum*) daily for seven days and was compared with a placebo group. Strikingly, all of the patients in the *Lactobacillus*-treated group were free of BV, as compared with only two patients without BV among the 16 placebo-treated women.[80]

Additional studies add to the body of evidence showing that supplementary probiotics may restore healthy vaginal flora.[81]

In a study reported in 2021, a product containing a strain of *Lactobacillus crispatus* isolated from the vagina of a healthy woman showed benefit in reducing recurrent BV when compared to a placebo group.[82]

Moreover, researchers observed that probiotics gradually restored vaginal microbial balance by suppressing the overgrowth of pathogens, yielding better long-term outcomes than the classic antibiotic (metronidazole) in treating BV.[83]

And in yet another study, this one over a 9-month period, 250 non-pregnant women with BV received either metronidazole or metronidazole followed by *Lactobacillus rhamnosus.* The latter group was more successful in preventing BV recurrence compared to the antibiotic-only group.[84]

One specific strain, *Lactobacillus rhamnosus* GR-1, is well documented for its urogenital health effects including a reduction in the recurrence of bacterial vaginosis.[85]

Importantly, the vaginal route is faster and more targeted than oral probiotics. A Table available online shows the effects of probiotic strains administered vaginally in clinical trials in reproductive and fertility-related disorders.[86] Though the use of vaginal probiotics is not widespread, the application shows promise. Probiotic supplements therefore may be beneficial. Several oral and vaginal probiotics containing *Lactobacillus* spp. are available on the market. Many of them may include one or more of these species: *L. crispatus, L. gasseri, L. plantarum, L. reuteri,* and *L. rhamnosus.* Strains of these species that are backed by clinical data should be used.

Probiotic therapy could be preferable as antibiotics have several disadvantages: antibiotic resistance, high rate of recurrent infections after treatment[87], and the clearance of microbes not targeted (collateral damage).[88]

However, the effectiveness of probiotics is not entirely certain.[89] Experts believe that perhaps a two-pronged approach is better: antibiotics to clear the infection followed by lactobacilli strains to repopulate.[90]

While there has been much research investigating the treatment of bacterial vaginosis and disordered microbiomes in optimizing outcomes in assisted reproductive technology (ART), the role of routinely prescribed probiotics is yet to be established. A 2020 meta-analysis in which only four articles were eligible for inclusion was disappointing in its breadth but is of interest and should spur more research.[91] One included study found that probiotics increased the clinical pregnancy rate non-significantly but also found a higher miscarriage rate in the group treated with probiotics. Also, any positive effect of probiotics on fertility does not show a clear separation line between males and females, as female infertility induced by an imbalance in the vaginal microbiome may affect the sperm parameters inside the female reproductive tract.[92]

In 2021, there was encouraging news.

A study of 44 women with reproductive failure compared to a control group (14 fertile women having at least two children after uncomplicated term pregnancies) using *Ligilactobacillus salivarius CECT5713* (formerly known as *Lactobacillus salivarius* CECT5713) had interesting results:[93]

- Lactobacilli detection frequency was much higher in the control group than in the infertile groups. The use of antibiotics in both infancy and adulthood was significantly higher among women in the infertile groups than among women in the control group.
- Seven species were identified in the samples from women of the control group: *L. crispatus* (the

dominant species), *L. jensenii, L. gasseri, L. Iners, Limosilactobacillus* (formerly *Lactobacillus*) *fermentum, L. salivarius*, and *Limosilactobacillus vaginalis.*

- However, the lactobacilli species profiles in the study groups were narrower than in controls and *L. fermentum, L. salivarius*, and *L. vaginalis* were not detected.
- The probiotic intervention modified key microbiological, biochemical, and immunological parameters in women who became pregnant. Daily oral administration of *L. salivarius* CECT5713 to women with reproductive failure for a maximum of 6 months resulted in an overall successful pregnancy rate of 56%.

A diagram available online in this study shows changes in vaginal parameters in women with a history of reproductive failure after the probiotic intervention according to their outcome (pregnancy versus no pregnancy). These factors include pH (acidity), Nugent score (mark of bacterial vaginosis), TGF-β 1, TGF-β 2, and VEGF concentrations (immunological activity), viable *Lactobacillus* counts and *L. salivarius* copies in cervicovaginal lavage samples.

The authors concluded: "The comparison between the vaginal microbiota of women with a history of reproductive failure, due to recurrent miscarriage or infertility, and healthy fertile women confirmed that dominance of specific species of lactobacilli in the vaginal microbiota plays a determinant role in the success of human reproduction."

In another area of research, polycystic ovary syndrome (PCOS) is observed to be marked by inflammation that may interfere with fertility. *Lactobacillus* strains have been shown to alleviate inflammation suggesting a role in the fertility of PCOS patients.[94]

Thus, *Lactobacillus* probiotic supplements, in restoring the healthy vaginal microbiota and suppressing inflammation, may lead to better fertility.

Prebiotics

Prebiotic: *A substrate that is selectively utilized by host microorganisms conferring a health benefit.*[95]

A number of fermentable carbohydrates can be prebiotic, provided that they are selectively utilized by the host microbiota and promote health.

One study of added fiber impact showed that partially hydrolyzed guar gum supplementation helped improve gut dysbiosis and the success of pregnancy in females with infertility.[96]

Fertility Takes Teamwork

A healthy vaginal microbiota depends on more than the woman. Sexual partners also must take responsibility. For example, semen may act as a medium for the transmission of microorganisms that may potentially become residents in the uterus.[97] Further studies are required to assess the role of this "seminovaginal" microbiome in couples' health, its alterations in infertility, and its consequences for the offspring.

One study conducted with 22 couples analyzed the effect of topical and oral antimicrobial therapy in both women with bacterial vaginosis and their male partners on vaginal and penile microbiomes. A reduction of bacterial diversity (a good thing) and a reduced abundance of taxa related to bacterial vaginosis in the vaginal microbiome were observed.[98]

Takeaway, So Far

Mounting evidence demonstrates the importance of reproductive tract microbiota in women's health and reproductive function.[99] Technological advances in the study of bacterial communities have enabled this valuable data.

Dysbiosis may not only be associated with infertility but may also play a role in IVF outcomes. Both men and women should be evaluated. The "seminovaginal" microbiome, meaning a functional unit able to influence not only the couples' health and their reproductive outcomes but also their offspring's health, is important.[100] To be clear, your microbiome offers a unique opportunity. Personalized treatment may lead to more and healthier pregnancies regardless of age or fertility status.

Impact of Female Obesity on Fertility

Obesity is surging globally. The numbers are especially alarming in the United States: 40% of women between the ages of 20 and 39 years are obese, according to 2018 data from the National Health and Nutrition Examination Survey.[101] As we shall see, obesity puts more than one-third of women at health risk in their prime reproductive years.

Obesity affects a woman's ability to get pregnant. The risk of infertility has been shown to be threefold higher in obese than in non-obese women, and several studies have demonstrated that obese females need a longer time to achieve pregnancy.[102]

Moreover, if pregnancy does occur, the stress and implications of obesity for the mother and her growing fetus are also negative. Complications include hypertensive disorders, gestational diabetes, preterm birth, and higher rates of cesarean delivery.[103]

The many ways obesity harms reproduction are becoming more clear:

Dysregulation of the Hypothalamic-Pituitary-Ovarian Axis (HPO Axis)

The hypothalamic-pituitary-ovarian (HPO) axis is a tightly regulated system controlling female reproduction. Obesity affects regulation of the HPO axis,[104] as evidenced in both animal[105] and human[106] studies. Female obesity is linked to abnormal menstrual cycles, infertility, reproductive wastage, and deficient hormone secretion.

Effects on the Oocyte

Recall that an oocyte is produced in the ovary by an ancestral cell and gives rise to the ovum or egg, which can be fertilized.

Much research indicates that obesity can harm the oocyte through a variety of perturbations.[107]

Even when obese women have normal menstrual periods or eumenorrhea (bleeding lasts 3-7 days, occurring every 21-45 days), they exhibit reduced fecundity.

Fecundity vs. Fertility

Fecundity is the physiological maximum potential reproductive output of an individual (usually female) over a lifetime. Fertility, on the other hand, is defined as the current (actual) reproductive performance of an individual.

Effects on the Preimplantation Embryo

Even if the oocyte is fertilized, obese women are more likely to create poor-quality embryos.

A study in overweight and obese women revealed that their embryos were less likely to develop after fertilization, and those that did showed reduced glucose consumption, modified amino acid metabolism and increased levels of triglycerides.[108]

Polycystic Ovary Syndrome Impact

As stated before, PCOS is a common but treatable endocrine disorder that is characterized by an excess secretion of testosterone hormone, elevation of inflammation, and ovarian dysfunction, all of which can lead to infertility.

Women with PCOS who are also obese demonstrate a more severe metabolic and reproductive phenotype. Obesity and/or PCOS-dependent changes to the gut microbiome contribute to ovarian inflammation, steroidogenesis and certain gene expression in the oocyte.[109] Because obesity is linked to inflammation, all mechanisms enrolled in oocyte differentiation and maturation including hormones, proteins and soluble factors released by adipocytes are deregulated and affected in their physiology.[110]

Actions of Adipokines

In addition to the hormone disorders and subfertility that are common in PCOS, adipocytes act as an endocrine organ in obesity. Adipose tissue releases a number of bioactive molecules called adipokines. These molecules interact with numerous metabolic pathways including oocyte differentiation and maturation.[111]

For example, altered levels of adipokines such as leptin can disturb the developing embryo.

Endometrium Impacts

The endometrium is the layer of the uterus in which the implantation of the fertilized egg takes place. If the implantation does not occur, the functional (outermost) layer of the endometrium is shed and expelled, leading to menstruation.

The cells of the endometrium undergo dramatic changes called decidualization in preparation for the pregnancy. Decidualization is essential for the establishment of a successful pregnancy. There is evidence that obese women show impairment of this crucial process. This may lead to placental abnormalities exhibited by higher rates of miscarriage, stillbirth, and preeclampsia in the obese population.[112]

High-Fat Diet Harms

A high-fat diet is a common cause of obesity.

Yet high dietary fat intake—even without obesity—impairs female hypothalamic-pituitary-ovarian axis functionality and fertility. How this occurs is complicated but appears to implicate increased leptin and insulin signaling, aggravated inflammation and other mechanisms.[113]

Weight and Assisted Reproductive Technology (ART)

Obese women have less success with in vitro fertilization.

Numerous studies have shown that a body mass index (BMI) that is too high is linked to a reduced probability of achieving pregnancy in women undergoing assisted reproductive technology (ART).[114]

From the start of IVF, obese women show higher levels of insulin, triglycerides, and markers of inflammation in follicular fluid.[115] Overweight and obesity are associated with negative outcomes for these patients due to their poor oocyte quality, as well as lower preimplantation rate and uterine receptivity.

A recent review cited research showing that during gonadotropin (a hormone secreted by the pituitary gland that affects the function of gonads or reproductive glands such as ovaries or testes) stimulation, higher doses and longer treatments are required for follicular development with lower oocyte yield. Moreover, oocytes that failed to fertilize in IVF cycles of morbidly obese women displayed multiple structure and functional alterations.[116]

How does BMI affect outcomes when ART is undertaken?

A recent analysis of 14,782 patients undergoing their first IVF at a single clinic in Xi'an, China is notable. Body weight and the IVF outcome of cumulative live birth rate (CLBR) illustrated an "inverted U shape" association. CLBR increased among underweight women, plateaued in normal weight and overweight women with a BMI* of 18.5–30.4, and then decreased in obese women proportionally to the accumulation of BMI. The study therefore may be useful for IVF patients with abnormal BMI to predict pregnancy outcome (CLBR) when attending weight counseling before initiating IVF cycles.[117]

*Note that a WHO expert consultation addressed the debate about the interpretation of BMI cut-off points for determining overweight and obesity in Asian populations. The WHO experts reported that the proportion of Asian people with a high risk of type 2 diabetes and cardiovascular disease is substantial at BMIs lower than the existing WHO cut-off point for overweight. However, no new cutoff points were defined.[118]

Current studies have adopted WHO classification criteria for BMI classification.

BMI, kg/m^2:

- Normal (18.5–24.9)
- Overweight (25.0–29.9)
- Obesity (≥30.0)

And finally, another study showed that weight gain in adulthood is negatively associated with ART success.[119]

Effect of Interventions

Researchers have asked whether weight loss would improve fertility and fecundity.

Results are mixed.

For example, a recent trial randomized more than 600 obese infertile women to either a 6-month lifestyle intervention before 18 months of infertility treatment or to immediate infertility treatment for 24 months. Notably, although the intervention group lost an average of 4.4 kg, it was bested by the group receiving prompt treatment in the primary outcome, which had a significantly higher vaginal birth rate within 24 months.[120]

However, in a cohort of 170 women undergoing IVF, short-term weight loss was associated with a higher yield of metaphase II oocytes in obese women, but clinical pregnancy rates and live birth rates (LBRs) were not affected. Still, overweight and obesity were associated with lower LBRs: 42% among women with a healthy BMI as opposed to 23% among overweight or obese women.[121]

Additional studies also showed that weight loss in women undergoing fertility treatments resulted in higher LBRs than those not losing weight.[122]

Of lifestyle interventions for encouraging healthier behaviors, all are likely to be cost-effective and appear to have positive effects on reproductive, maternal pregnancy, and birth outcomes, according to one study.[123]

A systematic review and meta-analysis of the effect of non-surgical weight loss strategies on fertility concluded with this advice: "Overweight and obese persons seeking fertility should be educated on the detrimental effects of fatness and the benefits of weight reduction, including improvement in pregnancy rates. A combination of a reduced calorie diet, by reducing fat and refined carbohydrate intake, and increased aerobic exercise should form the basis of programs designed for such individuals."[124]

Physical Activity

Independent of weight loss, physical activity in obese women undergoing fertility treatments has been shown to increase pregnancies and live birth rates. In a study of 216 obese infertile women, the chances to obtain a pregnancy and a baby were three-fold higher in the active obese infertile patients compared to the sedentary women.[125]

Moderate exercise may enhance fertility as it reduces systemic inflammatory mediators.[126] But too much of a good thing can hamper fertility. Extreme exercise can interfere with hormone levels and ovulation.

A 2021 study tracked exercise changes in 85 infertile women during confinement incurred by the COVID-19 pandemic. Not surprisingly, sitting increased while walking outdoors decreased. But as a group, vigorous and moderate exercise levels increased by 40 and 30%, respectively, despite the obstacles.[127]

Bariatric Surgery

In addition to diet and exercise, bariatric surgery (procedure on the stomach and/or intestines) may successfully reduce weight in obese women. Concerning however are an increased risk of small-for-gestational-age infants and a trend toward higher risks of stillbirth and neonatal death with no improvement in preterm birth, as seen in one study.[128]

Bariatric surgery does appear to improve the PCOS phenotype common in women with morbid obesity; lower androgen levels, resumption of regular menses, and improvement of metabolic parameters were observed.[129]

And in a 2021 meta-analysis of 10 studies with a total of 587 patients, bariatric surgery was a more effective treatment strategy for patients with PCOS and obesity compared to the medication metformin (a hypoglycemic drug used in the treatment of type 2 diabetes mellitus) alone. The pregnancy rate after bariatric surgery was greater than that for metformin.[130]

Weight loss programs through lifestyle modification in obese women have been proven to restore menstrual cyclicity and ovulation and improve the likelihood of conception.[131] Indeed, a recent review concluded that "lifestyle modifications prior to, and during ART have shown promise in enhancing fecundity."[132]

Impact of Low Female Weight on Fertility

Despite the current obesity epidemic, maternal underweight—especially globally—remains a fairly prevalent occurrence, troublesome because of potential adverse effects on fertility.[133]

Common causes of being underweight include disease, drug use, and energy deficiency as seen in some athletes (who expend much energy). Loss of fat tissue ensues; subsequent hormonal disturbances can lead to fertility problems.[134]

Ovarian dysfunction and infertility are often seen in women who are underweight and who have low amounts of body fat. Risk increased in women with a BMI below 17 in an early study of 597 women diagnosed with ovulatory infertility at seven infertility clinics. The risk though was slight compared to that in obese women.[135]

In addition, a meta-analysis of 78 studies, which included over one million women, found that the underweight women in developed countries had an increased risk of pre-term birth and low birth weight infants. In developing countries, underweight women showed an increased risk of low birth weight infants but not pre-term birth.[136]

Anorexia nervosa

A common cause of underweight status in women is anorexia nervosa (AN). Extremely low BMI is commonly seen in eating disorders such as AN, which usually strikes young women in their reproductive years. Note that other eating disorders like bulimia and binge eating are more apt to lead to obesity, also a problem in reproduction as described previously.

The prevalence of AN was recently estimated across a pool of 33 studies conducted from 1984 to 2017 with 315,877 participants across many countries. As expected, the disorder occurred differently when geography and gender were considered. In Western countries, the lifetime prevalence was 0.42% compared to 0.02% in Asian countries. Females had a 0.62% risk whereas males had only 0.04%.[137]

Although relatively uncommon, AN poses concerns regarding reproduction. Having a history of AN that is under control may not reduce fertility as was once thought; studies found that ability to get pregnant was equal to controls.[138] Nevertheless, a

2021 review of ten studies showed that rates of current and past eating disorders were higher among women seeking fertility treatment than in the general population.[139] One explanation may be that women with AN may be more likely to seek professional help prior to conception even though they do not appear to be at greater risk of infertility.[140]

Still, AN can negatively affect menstruation and maternal and fetal well-being. Many women with AN report disruptions in normal menstrual cycles which are most likely due to reduced estrogen levels induced by prolonged restriction of caloric intake and/or excessive exercise. Both the uterus and ovaries regress significantly after dramatic weight loss.[141]

Among 66 infertile women with amenorrhea or oligomenorrhea, 58% had eating disorders. But this finding included both anorexia nervosa and bulimia nervosa.[142]

Yet despite a high prevalence of menstrual irregularities, women with anorexia nervosa are becoming pregnant.

Based on a review of five studies including 353 women, if patients undergo eating-disorder treatment and weight restoration, it appeared unlikely that reproductive health was affected long-term by AN.[143]

One early review reported that past or recent AN does not appear to cause increased complications with most aspects of delivery including the risk of pre-term births, gestational hypertension/preeclampsia, induced labor, vacuum extraction, use of forceps, or breech presentation compared with the general population.

However, women with both recent and past AN were reported to have less gestational weight gain and babies with lower birth weights than the general population.[144]

Other eating disorders such as bulimia nervosa and binge eating disorder may not result in being underweight but do carry risks for the mother and child.[145]

The health of children into adulthood may be affected by a mother's eating disorder. Research on fetal programming reveals the serious consequences that AN may have on the long-term physical[146] and mental health of offspring.[147] Environmental processes influencing the propensity to disease in adulthood operate during the periconceptual, fetal, and infant phases of life.[148]

Undernutrition and overexposure to stress hormones are the main processes that underlie negative fetal programming. Notably, these are also the core features of AN.

Maternal malnutrition during pregnancy is linked to increased risk for metabolic diseases in adult offspring[149] and low birthweight infants are at increased risk for diminished cognitive function, behavioral problems, stress reactivity and psychopathology throughout their lifespan.[150]

Additionally, high levels of maternal anxiety during the prenatal period predict greater anxiety and cortisol stress response in offspring.[151]

Epigenetics (gene expression caused by mechanisms other than the genome) may explain the processes by which maternal nutrition and anxiety lead to long-term effects. Disturbingly, the effects are not limited only to immediate offspring but can be passed on to later generations. Grandchildren and beyond may be harmed.[152]

Women who are underweight when trying to conceive should take steps to gain weight by eating a more nutrient-dense diet as well as moderating any excessive exercise.

Part Three: Male Fertility and the Microbiome

It takes two to make a baby.

Yet in the archives of reproductive health studies, focus has traditionally been on a female's contribution. No surprise there. It may be understandable given the outsized role a woman's body plays in nurturing a fetus in its growth to a healthy newborn and on into a vigorous child.

But now we know that the male's role in that equation is substantial. Long considered a mere messenger of male DNA, seminal fluid provides components that allow the sperm to successfully reach and fertilize the egg (oocyte) and prepare the female immune system to tolerate the embryo.[153]

Semen is complex. It's a mixture of sperm and secretions of sexual accessory glands such as lipids, proteins, glycans and inorganic ions. Rich in nutrients, semen is an ideal environment for microbial growth.

Indeed, emerging evidence reveals that successful fertilization and development of the fetus depends on a healthy microbiome—in both partners.

The good news is that in principle there is no maximum age for fathering a child. There is no biological clock on a man's sperm. The not-so-good news? Sperm quality deteriorates as men age. Their testes tend to get smaller and softer, and sperm morphology (shape) and motility (movement) are likely to decline. In addition, there is a slightly higher risk of gene defects in their sperm.

Sperm Numbers, Shape, and Movement Matter in Fertility

Numbers (concentration) of sperm

Each time a man ejaculates, two to four milliliters (mL) of semen are released. Normal sperm concentrations range from 15 million to greater than 200 million sperm per mL of semen. Fewer than 15 million sperm per mL of semen is considered a low sperm count and can interfere with conceiving.

Shape (morphology) of sperm

The size and shape of sperm will also determine the likelihood of conception.

Movement (motility) of sperm

Swimming ability and a speed not seen as slow should be seen in more than 50% of sperm to be considered normal.

Derived from Greek roots, the biological terms for conditions of the sperm can be daunting. Fortunately, their meanings are fairly simple. This list will help you to decipher the language used in the many studies mentioned.

- *Aspermia*: Lack of semen
- *Hypospermia*: Semen volume below normal
- *Asthenozoospermia*: Reduced sperm motility
- *Oligozoospermia*: Low sperm count
- *Teratozoospermia*: Abnormal sperm shape
- *Oligoasthenozoospermia*: Combination of asthenozoospermia (reduced sperm motility) and oligozoospermia (low number of sperm)
- *Oligoasthenoteratozoospermia*: A condition that includes oligozoospermia (low number of sperm), asthenozoospermia (poor sperm movement), and teratozoospermia (abnormal sperm shape)

As with an army on a mission, these characteristics (number, shape and movement of sperm) are critical to success. First and foremost, healthy sperm are contingent on a healthy host.

Research on a man's health and the previously overlooked sperm is starting to trickle in. For instance, the unhealthy condition of obesity in reproductive-age men has nearly tripled in the past 30 years and coincides with an increase in male infertility worldwide. Obesity adversely impacts male reproductive potential not only by reducing sperm quality, but also by altering germ cells in the testes and ultimately mature sperm. The metabolic and reproductive health of offspring may also be impaired by male obesity. Health cues are transmitted to the next generation with the mediator mostly likely occurring via the sperm.[154] In addition, the importance of recognizing male infertility as a medical condition is seen in recent studies noting links between male infertility and future risks of testicular cancer, diabetes, and heart disease.[155] What's more, up to 30% of infertile men are labeled with idiopathic sperm abnormalities. This means that the cause is unknown.[156]

Disturbing news: In a span of about four decades (1973-2011), sperm concentration dropped more than 52% among random men in Western countries and the total sperm count dropped by 59%, according to a meta-analysis by Shanna H. Swan PhD and colleagues.[157] In her 2020 book Count Down,[158] Dr. Swan reveals that the rate of adverse changes—declining sperm counts and testosterone levels, testicular cancer increases and higher prevalence of erectile dysfunction—is increasing by 1% a year.

Based on two decades of research, Dr. Swan blames some of the damage on chemicals in our environment. The worst offenders are endocrine-disrupting chemicals but there are many. These chemicals that impair spermatogenesis include occupational exposure to persistent organochlorine pollutants (POPs), phthalates found in personal care products, and residues of pharmaceutical compounds in drinking water.

Dr. Swan sends a dire warning: "The current state of reproductive affairs can't continue much longer without threatening human survival."

Furthermore, if the decline continues, she predicts that by 2050, many couples will need to turn to technology to assist in reproduction.

Her book is a must-read for everyone but especially for those concerned about their own fertility or infertility.

Another way of assessing change in sperm quality over decades is by looking at the relative numbers of qualified potential sperm donors. As many as 60,000 children in the United States are conceived through sperm donation each year, indicating a big market for quality sperm. Alarmingly, sperm banks across the globe report that they are rejecting much higher percentages of donors. For example, the rate of qualified donors dropped from 56% in 2001 to 18% in 2015 at the Hunan Province Human Sperm Bank in China. The semen quality among young Chinese men has declined over 15 years, especially in terms of sperm concentration, total sperm count, sperm progressive motility, and normal morphology.[159]

Undeniably, infertility must be considered in light of both male and female factors. Both partners' reproductive systems join forces to create a baby.[160]

Lifestyle factors greatly impact the outcome. This is true whether you are trying to conceive for the first time or are seeking professional help after a year of attempts.

A nutritious diet, weight management, exercise, substance-free habits, stress reduction, and environmental toxin avoidance are all crucial to fertility, pregnancy and your future children.

And now add to the list: a healthy microbiome. This is welcome news. It adds another target—one which may be easier (and much cheaper) to address—for couples preparing and/or struggling to conceive.

The Role of Semen Microbiome on Reproduction

In the past, bacteria in semen were thought to be a sign of infection. Today, new technology has identified these organisms as an essential part of the environment.[161] Far from being interlopers, these microbes are in the right place. But their origins are not always clear. Scientists think they migrate from the urethra, gut, mouth, blood and a partner's vagina.

Taken together as a group, the set of organisms is called the microbiome. And it can be very different from one man to the next.[162]

Published in 2020, Microbiota and Human Reproduction: The Case of Male Infertility delves into how the semen microbiota impacts a man's health.[163] Significantly, evidence suggests a link between semen microbiome dysbiosis and infertility.

First, take a look at the many ways that microorganisms can impair spermatozoa functions:[164]

- Agglutination (clumping) of motile sperm
- Induction of apoptosis (programmed cell death)

- Production of immobilization factors
- Impairment of the acrosome reaction, a required step before the sperm fertilizes the egg

When organisms cause disease or illness to the host, they are considered pathogenic. Pathogens can cause inflammation (they are not the only cause) in the male genital tract. This inflammation is linked to poor semen quality, partially correlated with an increase in pathogens and a reduction in *Lactobacillus* strains.[165]

These disease mongers drive inflammation through a cascade of cytokines (signaling proteins of the immune system) or by enhanced production of reactive oxygen species (capable of causing damage to biomolecules). Oxidative stress ensues.

Oxidative stress: *An imbalance between the systemic manifestation of reactive oxygen species and a biological system's ability to readily detoxify the reactive intermediates or to repair the resulting damage.*

Current evidence links oxidative stress to male infertility, reduced sperm motility, sperm DNA damage and increased risk of recurrent abortions and genetic diseases. Sperm cells may be overwhelmed by these natural byproducts of oxygen during metabolism. Though numerous antioxidants are present in semen, including Vitamins A, E, C, and B complex, GSH, coenzyme Q10, carnitine, and minerals such as zinc, copper, selenium, and chromium, there may not be enough to avoid oxidative stress in some males.[166] More discussion of antioxidants appears in the supplement section of this book.

Oxidative stress can cause big problems. Some 30% to 80% of male sub-fertility may be associated with oxidative stress that damages spermatozoa. It can also reduce the success of in vitro fertilization (IVF) techniques.[167]

Escherichia coli (*E. coli)* are among the dominant bacteria isolated from the semen samples of males with infertility. E.coli inhibits spermatozoa motility in vitro and readily adheres to and agglutinates sperm.[168] In one study, a single incubation with *E. coli*, *Enterococcus fecalis*, and *Staphylococcus aureus* induced apoptosis (cell death) in human sperm.[169]

The most commonly detected sexually transmitted pathogen worldwide is *Chlamydia trachomatis.* The pathogen is linked with infertility.[170] Moreover, microbiota dysbiosis may increase the risk of *Chlamydia* infections. Women with bacterial vaginosis have a reduced presence of *Lactobacillus* spp.; after exposure to a male partner with chlamydial urethritis, a study observed a higher risk of *Chlamydia* infection.[171] Fortunately, the acidic (pH-lowering) impact of lactobacilli inactivates *Chlamydia.*[172]

A 2020 analysis was done of 55 observational studies with 51,299 subjects (collected between 1992 and 2019) to identify bacteria in the semen of infertile and fertile men:

Major findings:

The semen microbiome was rich and diverse in both fertile and infertile men. But the predominant bacteria were different. *Ureaplasma urealyticum, Enterococcus faecalis, Mycoplasma hominis* and *Prevotella* negatively impact semen parameters whereas *Lactobacillus* appears to protect sperm quality.[173]

Though antibiotics have traditionally treated these pathogens, increasing antibiotic drug resistance calls for alternate therapies. Correcting dysbiosis of the microbiota is a solution with potential for infertility.

Positive Effects of Lactobacilli

Lactobacilli appear to protect sperm quality. Not all strains though.

Certain strains of lactobacilli may have a protective role in the male genital tract, similar to what is seen in females. The transfer of microorganisms to the partner and offspring indicates that the seminal microbiome is important for the reproductive health of men, the health of the couple and the health of offspring as well.[174]

In one study, *Lactobacillus fermentum* L23 produced both preventative and curative effects on *E. coli* growth in a mouse model of vaginal tract infection.[175]

In another trial with mice, *Lactobacillus plantarum* 2621 overcame vaginal colonization and infertility induced by sperm-agglutinating *E. coli.* This particular strain of *Lactobacillus* was able to interrupt the dysbiotic impact of pathogens on fertility.[176]

Importantly, not all species act the same at all times. One such report suggested that *Lactobacillus iners* could either be health-promoting or implicated in dysbiosis and disease.[177] The mutable nature of some of these organisms makes forming recommendations more complicated.

Semen Microbes: Healthy or Not

Beyond looking at toxic microbes in infertility, scientists like to compare healthy semen donor samples alongside those with characteristics of infertility. Think of it as shooting for optimal conditions as opposed to merely avoiding disease or dysfunction.

For example, in one study which compared the semen microbiome of patients with prostatitis (inflammation of the prostate gland) versus healthy controls, a higher amount of lactobacilli, and in particular *L. iners*, was seen in the healthy subjects group.[178]

In the review Microbiota and Human Reproduction: The Case of Male Infertility, the authors assembled a concise list of microbial features in semen samples.[179] They stressed that these are correlations only and not conclusive or predictive of infertility:

- **Good-quality semen**: *Lactobacillus*
- **Low-quality semen**: *Anaeroccus, Bacteroides ureolyticus, Proteobacteria, Prevotella*-predominant

- **Azoospermic semen** (no sperm in a man's ejaculate): *Bacteroidetes* and *Firmicutes*

The semen microbiome appears to be vital to sperm quality. But the effects may be even more far-reaching. See, partners share microbes during sexual intercourse. Many of the bacterial taxa identified in semen also occur in the vaginal communities of some women, especially those with bacterial vaginosis, which suggests heterosexual sex partners may share bacteria.[180] Each partner can influence the microbiome composition of the other partner. How much influence varies with a host of factors: frequent sexual intercourse, multiple sexual partners, and uncircumcised male partners can alter vaginal microbiota and are linked to bacterial vaginosis.[181]

So we see that male and female microbiomes can engage. For example, microbiomes of semen and vaginal fluid (before and after intercourse) of 23 couples were profiled in a 2015 study. *Gardnerella vaginalis* in female partners was related to significant inflammation in male genital tracts. Also, the relative abundance of *Lactobacillus crispatus* decreased after intercourse, with a high consistency between semen and vaginal samples.[182]

In addition to influencing the vaginal microbiome, the semen microbiome may be able to overcome the cervical barrier and colonize the uterus. Microbes entering the uterus can cause infections and inflammation, which are linked to preterm birth, chronic lung disease and cerebral palsy.[183] A dysbiotic male microbiome is no small matter. The future health of children can be impacted.

Targeting the Seminal Microbiome

Probiotics

Probiotics are thought to enhance male fertility by improving sperm characteristics and testosterone levels.

Probiotics: Live microorganisms that, when administered in adequate amounts, confer a health benefit on the host.

The following trials in animals and humans illustrate probiotic effects:

A strain of *Lactobacillus rhamnosus* PB01 (DSM 14870) improved sperm quality parameters in obese mouse models.[184]

And a study with rats indicated that dietary probiotics had antioxidant activity and a protective effect against sperm damage induced by a high-fat diet.[185]

In a study in humans, *Lactobacillus rhamnosus* CECT8361 and *Bifidobacterium longum* CECT7347 improved sperm motility and reduced the percentage of sperm DNA fragmentation in asthenozoospermic (reduced sperm motility) males.[186]

In another study, a combination of three selected strains of lactobacilli (*Lactobacillus brevis CD2, L. salivarius FV2,* and *L. plantarum FV9)* used as vaginal tablets to treat bacterial vaginosis prevented sperm lipid peroxidation (oxidative deterioration) and preserved sperm motility and viability. Vaginal probiotic lactobacilli protected sperm from radical oxygen species in the presence of vaginal disorders. Simply put, the sperm had a better shot at fertilizing an egg.[187]

Because older men have falloffs in blood testosterone, some opt for supplemental hormones. But probiotics may be able to offset some of that decline. In one study with mice, *Lactobacillus reuteri* was able to sustain youthful levels as well as testicular size.[188]

Numerous fermented foods may contain probiotics but few are described adequately to be consistently reliable. For that reason, a probiotic supplement is often recommended.

Prebiotics

Prebiotic: *A substrate that is selectively utilized by host microorganisms conferring a health benefit.*[189]

Once again, many fermentable carbohydrates can be prebiotic, as long as they are selectively used by the host microbiota and promote health.

Prebiotics were able to ameliorate some semen parameters in both animal models and humans.[190]

Many foods and supplements provide much-needed prebiotics. Plants that are rich in prebiotics include onions, garlic, bananas, chicory root, and Jerusalem artichokes. Prebiotics added to foods or supplements include galacto-oligosaccharides (GOS), fructo-oligosaccharides (FOS), oligofructose (OF), chicory fiber, and inulin.

SYNBIOTICS

Synbiotic: A mixture comprising live microorganisms and substrate(s) selectively utilized by host microorganisms that confer a health benefit on the host.

A synbiotic of *Lactobacillus paracasei* B21060 with added prebiotics and additional ingredients over a period of 6 months improved sperm count and motility, and reduced the rate of atypical forms, in comparison to the control group. Testosterone levels were also improved.[191]

Supplement formulations often contain both probiotics and prebiotics. Read your labels.

This may be good news for infertility issues. These initial studies reveal that alterations to the male microbiota may enhance fertility.

Restoring male fertility with probiotics[192] may be enabled by:

- Reversing the impact of oxidative stress induced by a high-fat diet or old age
- Improving testosterone levels
- Improving sperm quality

New research suggests that ensuring a healthy seminal microbiome is an important step in health measures before trying to conceive. And know that making sure your microbiota is in good shape is recommended for all men—not just the infertile—who wish to optimize the health of their future child.

Other lifestyle changes are crucial too. Now, let's look at how another diet-related risk factor can interfere with male fertility.

Impact of Male Obesity on Fertility

Worldwide, obesity has nearly tripled since 1975. The United States is home to more than most countries: among younger men aged 20-39, 40% are obese according to 2018 data from the National Health and Nutrition Examination Survey.[193] Strikingly, this percentage matches that of women of the same age group, when reproduction is most likely.

As obesity rates soar, infertility is rising too.[194]

Is there a connection?

Past studies have suspected obesity as a factor in the decline in overall sperm quantity and quality in the last several decades.[195] Research observations included sperm concentration, motility and morphology as well as computed body mass index (BMI) for each patient. (BMI=kg/m^2):

- Normal (18.5–24.9)

- Overweight (25.0–29.9)
- Obesity (≥30.0)

Early on, contradictions were evident:

A 2010 review of 4,800 men across five studies found no correlation between BMI and sperm concentration and sperm count.[196]

Studies investigating paternal obesity and its effect on basic sperm parameters were summarized in a 2012 review. Sperm concentration appeared to be affected in a majority of studies but confounders such as lifestyle variables and self-reporting muddied conclusions.[197]

But then a year later, a review of 21 studies with 13,077 men reported an increased prevalence of oligospermia (low sperm count) or azoospermia (no measurable sperm) in both overweight and obese men.[198]

More studies have reported that increasing BMI negatively affects sperm parameters (volume, count and motility). Data collected from 4,440 men at three North American fertility clinics showed that unhealthy BMIs negatively impacted reproductive hormones, as expected, with the greatest absolute effect on the testosterone to estrogen (T/E) ratio, a common parameter of male sexual function. Also, all semen parameters were found to have negative correlations to BMI with significance noted for ejaculate volume, sperm concentration, morphology, and total motile count on multivariate analyses.[199]

And in another study published in 2020, the obese group within a 152 male cohort at an infertility clinic revealed significant deterioration of sperm quality; in particular, lower concentration and total number of spermatozoa in ejaculate and lower progressive motility.[200]

Thus the evidence appears to support that semen quality and quantity may suffer in obese men.

Mechanisms: How Does Obesity Do This?

Most likely in many ways.[201] It's nature's way of saying your baby deserves a healthy start. And a parent who can outrun a threat.

- Altered hormone levels. Testosterone naturally drops as men age. But obese men regardless of age will experience deficiencies of this hormone, which is crucial to successful reproduction.[202]
- Direct changes to sperm function and molecular composition
- Changes to DNA integrity[203]
- Shorter telomere (the natural end of a chromosome) length[204]
- Oxidative stress incurred by a high-fat diet and obesity can increase reactive oxygen species (ROS) impacting sperm quality.[205]

- Raised testicular temperature (the reason biking and hot tubs may be unfavorable)[206]
- Causing the gut to "leak" toxins, which drive inflammation in metabolic endotoxemia, a condition linked to reduced testosterone numbers.[207]
- In addition, obese infertile men typically eat a high fat, high sugar diet that in itself may cause reproductive impairment aside from excess adiposity.[208]

Obesity in Assisted Reproductive Treatment

When a couple seeks help via ART, outcomes appear to be different when the male is obese. Some research supports this:

- Odds of conceiving are lower.[209]
- Loss of pregnancy occurs more often.[210]
- Couples with an overweight man and normal weight female have increased time to conceive compared to couples with normal weight male partners.[211]

Obesity in the male should not be discounted; it appears to be every bit as detrimental to fertility and embryo health as it is in women.

Impact of Weight Loss

Researchers have tested whether weight loss in obese men would improve semen quality.

In a pilot study, 43 severely obese men with BMI > 33 kg/m^2 were followed through a 14-week residential weight loss program. The median weight loss was 15% and was associated with improved semen parameters, with the largest weight loss showing the best results.[212]

And in a 2018 study, adiposity demonstrated a significant relationship with DNA fragmentation and morphology, possibly contributing to subfertility in this population.[213]

Weight loss may improve metabolic health, which is linked to sperm function. A study in mice illustrates this. When glucose, insulin and cholesterol were returned to normal levels in high-fat fed mice with diet and exercise (regardless of adiposity), several improvements to sperm were observed: improved motility, morphology, molecular composition, and reductions in oxidative stress and DNA damage.[214]

However, a small study in obese men found that the dose of fat, not the type of fat, was unexpectedly the primary determinant of a post-meal decline in testosterone production.[215] In other words, monounsaturated fats (MUFA) or good fats (plentiful in avocados) may hypothetically have similar negative impacts on testosterone levels as polyunsaturated fats (PUFA) or so-called bad fats.

It appears that simple interventions may reverse the disease state that results in less than potent sperm. More research is needed.

Impact of Low Male Weight on Fertility

Obesity is not the only way in which weight can impact fertility in men. Being underweight can also cause problems. Unfortunately, most of the research in this vein has focused on underweight women with eating disorders.

However, a 2021 review summarized the evidence investigating links between male adiposity with sperm quality and reproductive hormones. The underweight category was associated with low sperm normal morphology.[216]

A healthy body weight is important for increasing sperm quality parameters and potentially male fertility.

Stress Effects

Apart from oxidative stress, the pressure of trying to conceive is added to the typical life stresses a man or woman might encounter on the road to being a parent.

Stress causes both physiological and emotional changes that can impact fertility.

One study of 1,215 men revealed that those with the highest stress levels (based on a questionnaire) had 38% lower sperm concentrations, 34% lower total sperm count, and 15% lower semen volume than those with intermediate stress levels.[217] Another study found a significant effect of age, obesity, mobile phone radiation and occupational stress on sperm DNA damage.[218]

Some evidence also links a history of exposure to psychological stress to higher rates of miscarriage among women.[219] Stress is a fact of life. Some people of course experience more than others. Whatever the level, stress must be managed. Getting instruction on how to handle stress or merely receiving support made a significant difference for women undergoing fertility treatment.[220] Whether through moderate exercise, meditation, probiotics, diet or similar therapies, stress should be reduced.

Tobacco, alcohol, marijuana, anti-depressants and other substances commonly used as stress relievers are not the answer. Instead, many studies suggest that they are part of the problem.

- Chemicals—over 4,000—in cigarettes can damage testosterone and harm sperm DNA, as well as reduce total sperm count, density, motility, volume and normal morphology. These chemicals also harm women. They can speed the rate at which a woman's eggs die and may lead to an increased risk of ectopic pregnancies, longer times to conception, and infertility in women who smoke.[221] Additionally, secondhand smoke increases the risk of miscarriage, stillbirth and ectopic pregnancy. Vaping and E-cigarettes may also do damage.[222] Adding insult to injury, the COVID-19 pandemic led to a 63% surge in tobacco consumption, according to one recent study, which tracked lifestyle habits of 85 infertile women during confinement. An increase in anxiety and depression levels was seen as possibly connected to the reported discomfort experienced by a large percentage of couples when fertility treatments were suspended because of the pandemic.[223]

- Marijuana is not a good substitute as it has been linked with sperm abnormalities.[224] Females who use marijuana are at an increased risk of primary infertility in comparison to non-users.[225]

- High alcohol intake may affect semen quality and testosterone production.[226] In women hoping to conceive, alcohol should be avoided completely. Fetal alcohol spectrum disorder is a common and devastating neurodevelopmental disorder.[227]

- Medications must also be scrutinized for damaging effects on reproductive health.[228] Antidepressants[229] and pain relievers[230]—even non-prescription types such as acetaminophen—have been linked to negative effects.

- Caffeine may be more likely to add to stress than relieve it. Then again, high amounts, as is likely when coffee or colas are drunk regularly, can be harmful to fertility. Miscarriage, spontaneous abortion, fetal death and stillbirth have been linked to caffeine consumption in recent research.[231]

Part Four: Fertility and Macronutrients

More than one in six couples struggle with infertility. We know that age is a big factor. Many other issues can be sources of problems: anatomical or genetic anomalies, systemic or neurological diseases, infections, trauma, and antibody development. And last but not least, an unhealthy lifestyle[232] and environmental toxins[233] can contribute to infertility.

Change the things you can change. The last two items fall into that category.

In light of increasingly delayed pregnancy,[234] finding alterable factors that affect the individual rates of reproductive decline is important. Diet is one such valuable target.

A healthy diet can prevent and treat a long list of ailments and diseases. The strong connection to a robust mind and body is unquestioned. Yet mystifyingly, many people regularly choose to eat high-fat, sugar-laden foods that are low in fiber, vitamins and minerals. Apparently, a daily medication—always with side effects—for reflux, high cholesterol, or high blood sugar is easier. Because of the popular consumption of sugary beverages, fast foods and processed foods as the main food groups in affluent countries, this unhealthy diet is referred to as a "Western diet."

Young women and men hoping to conceive a child may be unaware of the harms that such a diet may have on reproductive potential.

Diet Patterns

Fast food, delivery apps, food trucks, celebrated restaurants and a global migration of cuisines translate into a range of menus never before enjoyed in the history of humankind. Yet many people choose poorly.

A few studies address the broad concept of diet as it relates to conceiving a child.

Women

Based on a food questionnaire, women who ate large amounts of vegetables and fish had high rates of blastocyst formation. Recall that a blastocyte is a stage of embryo development. Red meat and alcohol correlated with lower rates of formation. In addition, aggressive dieting was linked to lower rates of blastocyst formation in a 2015 study.[235]

More recently, an ambitious cache of data has been made available through the Environment and Reproductive Health Study (EARTH).

In one application with 363 women seeking infertility care, dietary patterns were not linked to antral follicle count (AFC), a marker of ovarian reserve. Diminished ovarian reserve—the number and quality of eggs is lower than expected for age—is one of the major causes of female infertility.[236]

A diet widely considered beneficial to health is the Mediterranean Diet. The name is derived from the healthy meal regimens favored in the past by people living in Greece, Spain and Italy. Fish and poultry, plentiful fruits, vegetables, whole grains and olive oil with limited red meat and dairy products compose the diet. The diet is linked with positive changes in insulin resistance, metabolic disturbances, and the risk of obesity, all highly relevant when focusing on fertility.[237]

Recent data suggest that the Mediterranean Diet seems to preserve and improve fertility.[238]

One study showed that for those following a Mediterranean Diet, the live birth rate among non-obese infertile women under 35 years was 20% higher than among those using other diet types.[239]

Complications including gestational diabetes, low-birth weight, preterm delivery and hypertensive disorders of pregnancy were also reduced when a Mediterranean-style diet was consumed.[240]

Unfortunately, the COVID- 19 pandemic negatively changed diet patterns in 140 infertile women due to lockdowns imposed in Italy. There was a move away from the beneficial Mediterranean pattern with fruits, vegetables and legumes to a higher frequency of consumption of sweet pastries, cheese and meat. Snacking increased also, from 36% of women to 55% during lockdown.[241]

Another diet has been developed recently that specifically addresses fertility. The Pro-Fertility Diet is characterized by increased intake of whole grains, soy, seafood, dairy, low pesticide residue produce, along with supplemental folic acid, B_{12}, and vitamin D.

In one study, pretreatment adherence to the diet was associated with an increased probability of live birth in women undergoing in vitro fertilization and embryo transfer when compared to other dietary patterns.[242]

And a 2022 study found that increased compliance to the Pro-Fertility Diet was associated with improved markers of ovarian reserve in overweight and obese women (but not in normal weight women).[243]

The Pro-Fertility Diet may offer an extra level of benefit beyond that of the Mediterranean Diet for women seeking help with fertility.

An impressive trove of data on diet and its impact on fertility is available through the Nurses' Health Studies. Originated in 1976, the first cohort followed 121,700 married women through biannual surveys. The astonishing 90% response rate by these nurses over decades contributed greatly to public health. The studies have expanded through the years with additional cohorts.[244]

In 2016, in celebration of the 40th Anniversary of NHS, the *American Journal of Public Health's* September issue was dedicated to featuring the many contributions of the Nurses' Health Studies to public health.[245]

More than 17,000 women in one subset of the Nurses' Health Studies were surveyed on diet for eight years as they attempted pregnancy. They were assigned dietary scores based on their adherence to the "fertility diet" which is a pattern of dietary intake that has been linked with a lower risk of ovulatory infertility. The diet is characterized by less consumption of trans fats and animal protein and more consumption of low-glycemic carbohydrates, high-fat dairy, and multivitamins. Increasing adherence to a "fertility diet" pattern was associated with a lower risk of ovulatory disorder infertility. Notably, the authors suggested that the majority of infertility cases due to ovulation disorders may be preventable through modifications to diet and lifestyle.[246]

One exception to my no-anecdote rule is in order here. My mother Marcella Bradley Aigner was a dedicated participant in the first study. Her eight healthy children—the first six in a little over four years (two sets of twins)—surely informed the fertility data collection. She ate a healthy diet but obviously didn't require a gym for exercise.

Men

The Mediterranean Diet proved to be better in a study of 225 men in a fertility clinic in Athens, Greece. Better quality and quantity of sperm were linked to healthier food intake.[247]

A similarly healthful diet in Polish men was linked to increased sperm concentration, increased level of testosterone, and decreased percentage of sperm with DNA damage when compared to those eating a Western diet (red and processed meat, butter, high-fat dairy, refined grains, pizza, snacks, high-energy drinks, mayonnaise, and sweets).[248]

Additionally, when dietary patterns of young men were studied, it was reported that a diet rich in fruits, vegetables, chicken, fish, and whole grains may be positively associated with the percentage of progressively motile sperm.[249]

When 209 healthy young men in Spain were asked about diet, analysis identified two dietary patterns: a Mediterranean and a Western pattern. The Mediterranean Diet was positively associated with total sperm count. The Western Diet was positively related to the percentage of normal sperm but had a negative association with sperm concentration among overweight or obese men.[250]

A systematic review of 35 studies found that diets rich in omega-3 fatty acids, antioxidants, specific vitamins, and low in saturated fatty acids and trans-fatty acids were inversely related to low semen quality parameters. Diets rich in processed meat, soy foods, potatoes, full-fat dairy and total dairy products, cheese, coffee, alcohol, sugar-sweetened beverages and sweets were linked to poor quality of semen in some studies.[251]

A number of healthy dietary patterns may be of benefit. Healthy Eating Index, Dietary Approaches to Stop Hypertension, Alternate Mediterranean Diet Score and

Alternative Healthy Eating Index all linked with better sperm quality in 280 infertile men in a single-center study.[252]

Thus, semen quality appears better when foods eaten fall under the Mediterranean Diet or other healthy eating patterns and worse when a Western diet is ingested. But these studies didn't prove causation, only associations.

Couples

Additionally, one study looked at dietary patterns in 161 couples undergoing fertility treatments. Those following a Mediterranean Diet as opposed to a "health-conscious, low processed" diet had increased chances of pregnancy.[253]

It is clear. The Western diet is linked with reduced reproductive function while healthful diets improve them.[254]

PROTEINS

More than 10,000 proteins—made from twenty-plus amino acids—build muscle, bone, skin, hair, and essentially every other part of your body. Human needs are fairly straightforward. Adults should ingest a minimum of 0.8 grams of protein for each kilogram (2.2 lbs) of body weight per day. Intake of 1.0, 1.3, and 1.6 g protein per kg body weight per day is recommended for individuals with minimal, moderate, and intense physical activity, respectively. Long-term consumption of protein at 2 g per kg per day is safe for healthy adults.[255]

Estimated needs for pregnancy may vary depending on the stage.[256]

The source of protein is important: healthy protein sources like beans, nuts, low-fat dairy, fish, and poultry in place of red meat and processed meat can lower the risk of several diseases and premature death in humans.[257]

Ironically, protein is either maligned or celebrated these days. Vegan, gluten-free and Paleo diets—to name a few popular regimens—can upend ordinary patterns of protein intake, frequently among young people of childbearing ages. The effects of these diets on reproductive health are not clear.

However, several studies have looked at protein and its impact on reproductive health. Unfortunately, many variables such as genetics and lifestyle factors including exercise and smoking may cloud some conclusions.

Women

Research in animals suggests an adverse effect of a low-protein diet on prepubertal ovarian follicular number in offspring.[258] Limited research in humans also addresses the effect of protein on the participants' reproductive health. Researchers recently questioned if the amount and type of protein would affect a woman's follicles. In another EARTH study, 265 women undergoing fertility treatments filled out a food frequency questionnaire. Adjustments were made for age, body mass index, race, smoking status, and total energy intake. Total protein was unrelated to antral follicle count (the number of fluid-filled follicles detected using ultrasound). But infertile women with a higher intake (≥2.3 cups of milk/day) of dairy-derived proteins tended to have fewer antral follicles. The researchers hypothesized (informed guess) that bovine steroids and growth factors in milk or contamination by pesticides and endocrine-disrupting chemicals may upset the delicate dance of reproduction.[259]

The source of protein is increasingly seen as relevant. Animal protein has been linked to ovulation problems while plant proteins increased fertility in some age groups. It was noted that insulin response is lower with plant proteins than with animal proteins.[260]

Protein from animal sources may also disturb key androgens, which regulate ovarian function and female fertility.[261]

Dietary soy intake was positively related to the probability of having a live birth during infertility treatment with ART of 315 women.[262]

In addition, soy isoflavone supplements improved reproductive outcomes in IVF in one study.[263]

Men

One small study with nine overweight men revealed that proteins, particularly egg white protein, were beneficial in enhancing serum testosterone levels, with this effect observed within 4 to 5 hours after meal consumption.[264]

In another trial, soy protein effects were assessed for 99 male partners of subfertile couples. The data suggested that a higher intake of soy foods and soy isoflavones was associated with lower sperm concentration but was unrelated to sperm motility, sperm morphology or ejaculate volume. Isoflavones are plant-derived polyphenolic compounds with estrogenic activity. The fact that they are found mainly in soybeans and soy-derived products suggests that may be a factor in soy's influence on sperm concentration.[265]

Carbohydrates

Carbohydrates get no respect. Some weight loss diets try to eliminate them almost entirely. A better decision would be based on the type of carbohydrate and not the amount. To be sure, cookies, cakes and potato chips are carbohydrate-rich but are usually made from unhealthy simple sugars and starches packed with saturated fats. Instead, whole grain breads and grains supply needed nutrients and fiber to your body. And what are those rock stars of good nutrition—fruits and vegetables—if not rich in carbohydrates?

Carbohydrates are structurally diverse: they include monosaccharides such as glucose, fructose, and galactose; disaccharides such as sucrose and lactose; and polysaccharides such as starch and dietary fiber. Artificial sugars are also increasingly added to foods and beverages.

The unique structures of carbohydrates determine their specific actions in the body. For example, different types of carbohydrates affect blood sugar differently. Both the quality and quantity of carbohydrates in diet influence glucose metabolism, affecting insulin demand or sensitivity in healthy individuals. Why is this relevant? Both insulin sensitivity and glucose metabolism can significantly affect ovulation and female fertility.

Fortunately, nutrition science has developed tools to quantify the effect of carbohydrates in the diet on blood glucose.

The glycemic index assigns a numeric score (1 to 100) to a food based on how insignificantly (1) or drastically (100) it makes your blood sugar rise. Generally, processed foods have higher scores whereas foods with fiber and fat score lower as they slow the blood sugar spike. The total carbohydrate in a portion of food must also be considered. Both the quality and quantity of carbohydrates in any given food are taken together to arrive at what is called the glycemic load. A healthy fruit like watermelon may score an 80 on the glycemic index but with its low carbohydrate content supplies a mere glycemic load of five.[266]

A high score is not the goal here.

A list of the glycemic index and glycemic load for more than 100 common foods is available online at https://extension.oregonstate.edu/sites/default/files/documents/1/glycemicindex.pdf

Women

High glycemic index and load have been associated with higher fasting glucose concentrations, hyperinsulinemia, and insulin resistance, and therefore higher concentrations of insulin-like growth factor I (IGF-I) and androgens. Such issues can lead to endocrine disturbances, which in turn may alter the maturation of oocytes.[267]

Indeed, data from the Nurses' Health Study II indicated that greater carbohydrate intake and dietary glycemic load were associated with an increased risk of infertility as a result of ovulation disorders.[268]

Other studies also found that higher consumption of high glycemic index products and carbohydrates was related to lower chances of becoming pregnant.[269]

In research from the EARTH study, women undergoing IVF with a higher intake of whole grains achieved increased implantation and live birth success rates. Whether this was due to micronutrient or estrogen content of whole grains or perhaps through improved glucose metabolism was not clear.[270]

Refined sugar and artificial sweetener intake in women may also have a negative effect on ART success. Higher intake of sugared soda was associated with lower total, mature, and fertilized oocytes and top-quality embryos after ovarian stimulation in a prospective study of 340 women undergoing IVF.[271] Analysis of food frequency data of 524 women showed that consumption of ≥3 servings of regular soft drinks or any amount of diet soft drinks was linked with oocyte dysmorphism, diminished embryo quality on days 2 and 3 of culture, and a mild effect on blastocyst formation, implantation and pregnancy rate. Consumption of artificially sweetened coffee was negatively associated with embryo quality on days 2 and 3.[272]

Men

Several studies suggest a negative association between sugar and semen quality.[273] Sweetened beverages in one study were linked to reduced sperm motility in healthy young men, possibly due to insulin resistance and oxidative stress.[274]

In a study looking at macronutrient effects on testosterone levels in overweight and obese men, carbohydrates—in the form of orange juice—alone had little effect on levels.[275] But an earlier study observed that a glucose load induced a reduction in total and free testosterone levels in men.[276]

Other High Carbohydrate Foods

As mentioned, high carbohydrate foods like fruits and vegetables are sometimes shunned or even eliminated in trendy diets. But research shows that a higher intake of both consistently links to better sperm motility and morphology in men seeking fertility assistance in clinics.[277]

A 2021 study in 90 healthy men showed that high fruit and vegetable consumption (ascertained by a 3-day food recall) was positively correlated to sperm quality parameters.[278]

Other carbohydrate-rich foods such as whole grain breads, grains and cereals supply needed fiber, vitamins and minerals; for all populations, they are much preferred to products made with refined grains.

FATS

Fats store energy and are crucial for numerous functions and reactions in the body. Like carbohydrates, they are often maligned but always prominent in Western diets.

Fats are made of fatty acids. Depending on their source, fats impact health quite differently. Animal foods contain large amounts of saturated fatty acids, while both animal and plant sources supply unsaturated fatty acids.

Saturated fats

FYI: Saturated fats are so-called because they have no double bonds between carbon molecules. The carbon molecules are already "saturated" with hydrogen molecules and are solid at room temperature.

Saturated fats are mainly found in animal foods—think butter, ice cream, and hamburgers—and also in a few plant foods such as coconut, coconut oil, palm oil, and palm kernel oil.

In women, high dietary fat intake including saturated fats is associated with changes in reproductive function, including menstrual cycle length, reproductive hormone levels, and embryo quality in assisted reproductive technology cycles.[279]

In a dose-response study of 701 young Danish men from the general population, a lower sperm concentration and total sperm count were found in men with a high intake of saturated fat.[280]

Among 99 men attending a fertility clinic, a high intake of saturated fats was negatively related to sperm concentration whereas a higher intake of omega-3 fats was positively related to sperm morphology.[281]

Trans fats

Trans fats are hydrogenated vegetable oils, ubiquitous in margarine and shortenings at one time but now are being removed from the food supply of many but not all countries. Manufactured trans fats are the worst type of fat for the heart, blood vessels, and blood sugars.

In regards to fertility issues, these proinflammatory fats have been linked to a higher risk of insulin resistance, PCOS and endometriosis.[282]

In another study, 33 men undergoing infertility evaluation provided semen samples for fatty acid composition analysis. A notable finding was that trans fatty acids were present and were inversely related to sperm concentration.[283]

Still found in many countries' food supplies, banned trans fats can increase inflammation and increase insulin resistance, impacting fertility.[284] Read your labels.

Unsaturated fats

FYI: Unsaturated fatty acids have one or more double bonds. The litany of types sounds like fraternity row at a university. The most common omega-3 fatty acids are alpha-linolenic acid (ALA), eicosapentaenoic acid (EPA) and docosahexaenoic acid (DHA); the most common omega-6 fatty acids are linoleic acid (LA), dihommo-gamma linolenic acid (DGLA) and arachidonic acid (AA). Both omega-3 and omega-6 fatty acids are "essential." This means they are required for human health but the body cannot make them. You must get these essential fatty acids through food or supplements. Omega-9 fatty acids such as oleic acid can be made by the body but are also found in foods.

There are two categories of "good" unsaturated fats: Polyunsaturated fats (PUFAs) and monounsaturated fats (MUFAs). First, we will look at the evidence regarding PUFAs.

Polyunsaturated fats *(PUFAs) are long chains with two or more double bonds between the carbon atoms. Omega-3 and omega-6 predominate and come from both plant and animal sources. PUFAs are found in high concentrations in sunflower, corn, soybean, and flaxseed oils, walnuts, flax seeds, cold-water fish and canola oil.*

The recommended ratio of omega-6 to omega-3 fatty acids in the diet is 4:1 or less (primitive humans boasted 1:1). The Western diet has a ratio between 10:1 and a whopping 50:1. A steady diet of fast foods and processed foods feeds into that lopsided ratio. A lower ratio is linked to a lower risk of many chronic diseases and may also be associated with fertility and reproductive health.[285]

Both omega-3 and omega-6 fatty acids can influence reproductive processes through a variety of mechanisms. Because of the need to balance the aforementioned unhealthy ratio, much of the research has focused on omega-3 fatty acids in diet and supplements.

From a review of studies in animals, dietary supplementation with omega fatty acids not only impacted prostaglandin and ovarian steroid synthesis but also improved folliculogenesis, oocyte maturation and ovulation, embryo quality and implantation, placentation and the female reproductive lifespan.[286]

Women

Omega-3 fatty acids are well known for their benefit to heart health. They have also been studied in relation to fertility and reproduction. On the one hand, their anti-inflammatory properties may assist fertility but some studies with infertile women don't show a benefit.[287]

Also, in a 2020 study with 200 women with no history of infertility, there was no strong association between serum concentrations of omega-3 and the probability of conceiving naturally.[288]

Notably, among women of normal but not obese weight, omega-3 supplementation reduced follicle-stimulating hormone, an outcome that may be of benefit for those with diminished ovarian reserve.[289]

Intake of omega-3 fatty acids improved embryo quality and implantation rates in both humans and animals, as seen in a review of research conducted over the last decade.[290]

Also, results of fatty acid analysis in the 2018 Earth study showed that patients who consumed food rich in docosahexaenoic acid (DHA) and eicosapentaenoic acid (EPA) omega-3 fatty acids and who also had high blood concentrations were more likely to have successful ART outcomes. In addition, EPA was reported to be linked to high live birth rates when its concentration was high.[291]

Men

Dietary fats affect sperm lipid membrane composition, a key structure influencing the function of sperm.[292]

Intake of fish oil supplements was associated with higher semen volume and total sperm count, larger testicular size, and other functional markers in a cross-sectional study of 1679 young men in Denmark. Actual amounts and types of fatty acids were not known.[293]

In Spain, a smaller group of 209 healthy males completed questionnaires on lifestyle, diet, and smoking and then underwent physical and blood examination. Fatty acid consumption influenced testicular function with diverse effects from different types: intake of omega-3: positive effects; omega-6: variable effects; trans fatty acids: negative effects.[294]

Monounsaturated fats

Monounsaturated fats (MUFAs) also merit attention in fertility and birth outcomes.

Monounsaturated fats (MUFAs) are a type of unsaturated fat with only one double bond. They are found in high concentrations in olive, peanut and canola oils, as well as avocados, nuts and seeds. Omega-9 fatty acids are generally monounsaturated.

These fats (especially oleic acid) make up a large portion of the blood of newborn infants from healthy mothers.[295] Congenital birth defects in one small study were lower when the maternal diet was rich in oleic acid.[296]

Based on a large cohort in the Nurses' Health Study II, researchers found that consuming just 2% of energy from unprocessed MUFA instead of hydrogenated trans fats was associated with less than half of the risk of ovulatory infertility.[297] One explanation may be that these fats can bind with the peroxisome proliferator-activated receptor γ (PPAR-γ), thus decreasing inflammation and positively affecting fertility.

When studied in women undergoing IVF, greater intakes of MUFA were related to nearly three and half times higher odds of live birth after embryo transfer, compared to lower intakes.[298] (Paper is nested in the conference report.)

Another study showed a positive correlation between preconception levels of MUFA in women and fertility and time to achieve pregnancy.[299]

And finally, a review of the literature from Poland suggested MUFA can help to improve a woman's fertility, while the intake of trans fats should be avoided.[300]

Specific Foods

The main effects of specific foods on semen quality and potential mechanisms are summarized in a Table available online.[301] Let's take a look at the worst offenders.

Meat

Beef, lamb, and pork are all high in saturated fat. Even lean cuts of beef contain 4.5 grams of saturated per 100-gram serving. As documented before, a high saturated fat intake is linked to lower sperm concentration and total sperm count.

A recent review also noted the dangers of processed meats. Curing (preserving with salt) especially can create nitrates, which can damage DNA in sperm (as well as cause cancer). Some evidence shows an association between processed red meat consumption and decreased sperm counts and altered sperm motility.[302]

Asthenozoospermia (reduced sperm motility) has been linked to processed meats with high saturated fats.[303] Another study observed that processed meat intake was negatively associated with fertilization rates among 141 couples undergoing conventional IVF.[304]

Avoiding hot dogs, sausage, bacon, beef jerky and cold cuts is advised. Also, grilling red meats at high temperatures can produce harmful compounds.

Eating organ meats including liver from beef, calf, pork, chicken, and turkey appeared to be beneficial for various sperm parameters in both healthy young men and those seeking fertility help according to one comprehensive review. Chicken meat was not related to sperm parameters.

The impact of fish intake was also studied but the results were inconsistent.[305] However, one study showed that greater male and female seafood intake was associated with a shorter time to pregnancy.[306] Mercury content of fish is a concern for pregnant women. A risk-benefit evaluation paper concluded that consumption of fish species with a low mercury concentration and high concentrations of DHA + EPA and ω-3 PUFA (e.g., salmon, mackerel, and amberjack) are recommended.[307]

Dairy Products

Dairy products have been a rich source of fats (as well as protein, carbohydrates and micronutrients) since 7000 years BC when the people in Anatolia (now Turkey) tapped the milk of goats and cattle.[308] Today, dairy products including yogurt and milk can be processed to eliminate most saturated fats.

In healthy young men in one study, full-fat dairy foods were linked with lower percent progressively motile spermatozoa.[309]

When dietary intake of a group of men at a fertility clinic was studied, the findings suggested that low-fat dairy intake, particularly low-fat milk, was related to higher sperm concentration and progressive motility, whereas cheese intake was related to lower sperm concentration among past or current smokers.[310]

And intake of skim milk was associated with a lower risk of asthenozoospermia in another study.[311]

Therefore, full-fat dairy products appear to be detrimental to sperm parameters whereas low-fat ones are beneficial. According to one broad review, numerous studies show the damaging effect of fat (total or saturated) on sperm count and sperm concentration.[312]

A recent study on obese men found that the dose of fat, not the type of fat, was the primary determinant of a post-meal decline in testosterone production. Surprisingly, MUFA-rich olive oil had a similar negative impact on serum testosterone levels as that of plant-based polyunsaturated fatty acids or animal-based saturated fats.[313]

Conversely, full-fat dairy may increase fertility in women. One study showed that the consumption of low-fat dairy—including low-fat milk, yogurt, and cottage cheese—increased the risk of infertility due to anovulation, whereas high-fat dairy increased fertility.[314] However, later studies did not confirm this effect.[315]

Part Five: Fertility and Micronutrients

Vitamins and Minerals

Valuable things come in small packages. Micronutrients including vitamins and minerals are required for normal function. Many are also designated "essential"; a term which when used in this context means that the body needs an external source.

FYI: Recommended Dietary Allowance (RDA) is the average daily level of intake sufficient to meet the nutrient requirements of nearly all (97%-98%) healthy people.[316]

Vitamins

Water-soluble: Vitamin C, thiamin (B_1), riboflavin (B_2), niacin (B_3), pantothenic acid (B_5), pyridoxal (B_6), biotin (B_7), folate/folic acid (B_9) and cobalamin (B_{12}).

Fat-soluble: Vitamins A, D, E and K

Minerals

A large number of minerals are essential for health including calcium, phosphorus, potassium, sodium, chloride, magnesium, iron, zinc, iodine, sulfur, cobalt, copper, fluoride, manganese, silicon, nickel, chromium, lithium, molybdenum, and selenium.[317] Some are required in gram measures while for others a microgram or so will do.

All micronutrients are important for the general health of any human being. Future parents need more.

Much evidence shows that there is an increased need for vitamins and minerals (as well as energy and other nutrients) to support healthy pregnancies and healthy babies. Eating for two not only means extra calories but also more micronutrients. The fetus depends entirely on the mother for its nutrition.

Nutrient-dense foods should prevail. Hint: Soda and fries are not in that category. The Dietary Guidelines for Americans 2020-2025 recommend nutrient-dense forms of foods and beverages across all food groups, in recommended amounts, and within calorie limits.

"Nutrient-dense foods and beverages provide vitamins, minerals, and other health-promoting components and have little added sugars, saturated fat, and sodium. Vegetables, fruits, whole grains, seafood, eggs, beans, peas, and lentils, unsalted nuts and seeds, fat-free and low-fat dairy products, and lean meats and poultry—when prepared with no or little added sugars, saturated fat, and sodium—are nutrient-dense foods."[318]

For more information about building a healthy dietary pattern, see the Dietary Guidelines for Americans[319] and the U.S. Department of Agriculture's MyPlate.[320]

When an optimum diet is not eaten, micronutrient status may suffer. It is well established that serious reproductive problems can arise from micronutrient deficiencies: Pre-eclampsia, preterm deliveries, neural tube defects of the brain or spinal cord (such as spina bifida), and other congenital abnormalities as well as low birthweight.[321]

Deficiencies can cause severe problems:

- Calcium deficiency is linked to the development of pre-eclampsia, a hypertensive disorder in pregnancy.[322]
- Iron deficiency—extremely common in women—causes anemia and impairs brain development in the infant. A greater risk of preterm birth, low birth weight or small-for-gestational-age infants are also observed.[323]
- Low copper in early pregnancy is a risk factor for spontaneous abortion and central nervous system malformations.[324]
- Iodine deficiency is strongly associated with hypothyroidism in mothers and infants. Iodine deficiency is the leading cause of preventable intellectual disability worldwide.[325]
- Magnesium deficiency is strongly associated with an increased risk of preeclampsia and preterm labor.[326]

- Low levels or unusually high levels of manganese are a problem for fetal growth, neurodevelopment, and psychomotor development.[327]
- Low chromium levels are associated with gestational diabetes.[328]

Once again, these are micronutrients, needed only in tiny amounts. Even so, it can be hard to get enough through diet. What's more, these needs are not static. As the pregnancy progresses, many levels of vitamins and minerals become depleted. Supplementation may be necessary for deficient or high-risk individuals during pregnancy. For that reason, prenatal vitamin and mineral supplements are often recommended even before the planning stages of pregnancy. But they have to be calibrated. Excess amounts can cause problems for the mother and child. Choosing a proper prenatal supplement is all-important.

Which prenatal supplement is best?

Though the FDA has RDAs for total vitamin/mineral intake from food and supplements, it has not established recommendations for prenatal supplements. Unfortunately, there is wide variation in the content and quality. A 2021 review found that "approximately 44% of prenatal supplements (83 out of the 188 evaluated) consist of only a single pill with limited amounts of vitamins and often few or no minerals. This results in insufficient vitamin/mineral supplementation for many women and, hence, does not adequately protect them, or their children, from pregnancy complications and infant health problems."[329]

For example, the review reports that although most supplements contained some iron, zinc, and calcium, other essential minerals were included at a lower rate. And when minerals were included, most dosages were below recommended levels.

Considering the high stakes, special attention should be paid to choosing these supplements. Consult a dietitian or doctor about which formula is right for you. The Prenatal Rater app from the Neurological Health Foundation can also help you choose from the hundreds of products on the market.

While pregnancy needs are of utmost importance, the focus of this book is on fertility, which may require different levels of vitamins and minerals.

Micronutrients and fertility

Much less is known about how deficiencies may impact fertility. But we have ample evidence that micronutrients have vital roles at various stages integral to fertility.[330]

A few of the many examples (expanded on later):

- *Folate*: oocyte quality, maturation, fertilization, and implantation
- *Zinc*: ovulation and the menstrual cycle

- *Vitamin A*: oocyte quality and blastogenesis (development of the embryo)

And yes, lower than recommended levels of certain micronutrients have been reported in women who are diagnosed as infertile. The research is detailed in this section. Studies suggest that supplementation with micronutrients may assist in fertility in both healthy and infertile women. According to one review, micronutrient supplementation had a small but beneficial effect on fertility in healthy and infertile women, including a shorter time to pregnancy and an increased chance of becoming pregnant.[331] By restoring levels to recommended levels and reducing oxidative stress, fertility may be enhanced. Men too may be at risk as the studies show.

Specific micronutrients are getting attention (and research money) for their involvement in fertility. Deficiencies of copper, iodine, magnesium, manganese, molybdenum and others may also cause problems with pregnancy, birth and offspring but solid links to fertility have not been made. Stay tuned.

This book focuses on the likely operatives.

First, take a look at antioxidants and the power they wield in fertility.

ANTIOXIDANTS

Cells convert nutrients to energy through oxidative reactions. Molecules such as reactive oxygen species (ROS) are produced, which is normal cell function. But when ROS gets excessive, an imbalance called oxidative stress ensues, bringing a cascade of problems. Fortunately, certain compounds—called antioxidants—can neutralize these effects. Antioxidants prevent the damage to cells and DNA from oxidative stress.

What upsets the balance? Excessive ROS production (which can occur with tobacco, recreational drugs, alcohol use, extremes of body weight, exposure to environmental toxins, and advanced maternal age) or when antioxidant reserves within the body are low.[332]

Oxidative stress can lead to infertility and conditions that may reduce fertility, such as polycystic ovary syndrome (PCOS) and endometriosis. Complications such as spontaneous abortion, recurrent pregnancy loss, and preeclampsia, can also develop.[333]

Oxidative stress can impair physiological female reactions such as oocyte maturation, ovulation, luteolysis, and follicle atresia. Antioxidants protect DNA and other vital molecules against oxidative damage that would otherwise induce apoptosis (death of cells).[334]

What's more, oxidative stress may be associated with infertility of both known and idiopathic (unknown) origins.[335]

In men, oxidative stress is well known for its harm to fertility. Antioxidants show potential in the treatment of male infertility.[336]

Reducing oxidative stress in both men and women is paramount when planning a pregnancy. Fortunately, you can play a big part in reaching this goal by changing your lifestyle and diet.

Two ways:

Eliminate the causes of excessive ROS that are controllable: tobacco, recreational drugs, alcohol, excess weight or too little weight for height, and environmental toxin exposure. Age is obviously one factor that you cannot change.

Eat a healthy diet. Reams of research over decades confirm that a healthy diet is one rich in fruits, non-starchy vegetables, nuts, legumes, fish, vegetable oils, yogurt, and whole grains; and fewer red meats, processed (sodium-preserved) meats, and foods higher in refined carbohydrates and salt. Diets bountiful with fruits and vegetables are known to reduce the risk of obesity, metabolic syndrome, type 2 diabetes, cardiovascular disease, inflammation, neurological disorders, and cancer.[337]

Plants are particularly abundant in compounds with antioxidant properties. These include polyphenols, carotenoids, capsaicinoids and casinoids, isothiocyanates, and catechins. Many have been explored for roles in prevention and/or treatment of disease.[338]

Women

In a pilot study, an antioxidant multi-nutrient supplement given after in vitro fertilization (IVF)/intracytoplasmic sperm injection (ICSI) resulted in a higher proportion of women with at least one good-quality embryo compared with folic acid only.[339]

In another study, more good-quality oocytes were retrieved when micronutrients were started three months before IVF cycles. The treatment protected the follicular fluid and serum proteins from oxidative damage.[340]

Antioxidants may have different effects, depending on the body mass index (BMI) and age of the supplemented women, as reported in 2014 research.[341] The research suggests that increased intake of antioxidant vitamins may shorten the time required to achieve pregnancy. Both a woman's age and weight impacted results:

- A shorter time to pregnancy (TTP) occurred with increasing β-carotene and vitamin C in women younger than 35 years. In older women over age 35, vitamin E showed positive effects.
- Shorter TTP was observed among women with variations in effect when weight was considered. In women of normal weight, increasing vitamin C resulted in shorter TTP; in overweight women, increasing β-carotene resulted in a shorter TTP.

Increased antioxidant intake may make pregnancy happen faster. Supplements may be recommended when diet alone doesn't meet needs.

Several studies report links between achieving pregnancy and the use of a nutritional supplement containing multiple vitamins and minerals:

In a small pilot study, one-third of supplemented women became pregnant compared with none in the group that received a placebo.[342]

A later study with a larger group of women seemed to confirm the benefit: after 3 months, 26% of women in the supplemented group were pregnant compared with none in the placebo group, whereas another 32% conceived after 6 months of supplement use.[343]

But not all studies assessing the effects of antioxidants on fertility have had positive results.

In a 2020 meta-analysis of 63 trials involving 7,760 women, there was low- to very low-quality evidence to show that taking an antioxidant may benefit subfertile women. Researchers compared oral antioxidants, including combinations of antioxidants, N-acetylcysteine, melatonin, L-arginine, myo-inositol, carnitine, selenium, vitamin E, vitamin B complex, vitamin C, vitamin D+calcium, CoQ10, and omega-3-polyunsaturated fatty acids versus placebo, no treatment/standard treatment or another antioxidant.[344]

Nevertheless, some of these results suggest that the use of a supplement in women susceptible to micronutrient deficiencies may help optimize their reproductive health.[345]

Men

It is widely accepted that oxidative stress plays a role in the pathophysiology of male infertility and that antioxidants could have a role in the treatment of male infertility.[346]

Oxidative stress may reduce sperm quality,[347] a major cause of male infertility.[348]

Moreover, evidence suggests that men with a high dietary intake of antioxidants have a lower frequency of sperm aneuploidy (having one or a few chromosomes above or below the normal chromosome number) and improve sperm quality.[349]

Indeed, sperm oxidative stress correlated with decreased sperm motility, increased sperm DNA damage, decreased acrosome reaction and lower embryo implantation rates following IVF.[350]

A 2021 study reported that 30% to 80% of male sub-fertility may be associated with oxidative stress that damages spermatozoa and can decrease the success of in vitro fertilization (IVF) techniques.[351]

Though numerous antioxidants are present in semen, including Vitamins A, E, C, and B complex, glutathione, CoQ_{10}, carnitine, and minerals such as zinc, copper, selenium, and chromium, there may not be enough to avoid oxidative stress in some males.[352]

One recent trial evaluated the dietary intake of 175 oligoasthenospermic (low sperm count) men via a detailed food frequency questionnaire. Results showed an inverse association between dietary consumption of some antioxidants and sperm-related parameters.[353]

Let's take a closer look at specific micronutrients—most with antioxidant activity—that have been researched in connection to fertility and reproductive health. There are probably more, many more; the symbiosis of plants and animals is complicated and scientists have not unraveled all its mysteries. Not even close.

Be aware that Vitamins D, B_6, B_{12} and folate may also have antioxidant capacity in addition to the specific actions reported most often pertinent to reproduction.

Food sources and information about supplements are included. Be cautious. Many of these when given in supplement form may interact with medications in harmful or dangerous ways.

The United States National Institutes of Health (NIH) Office of Dietary Supplements provides comprehensive information on most of these supplements including their roles in health, metabolic activity, deficiencies, toxicities, recommended intakes, upper limits, and medication interactions.[354] When appropriate, this source informs the evidence I have included here. I sought data on both women and men, both unquestionably germane to the discussion. But at times, available research on a micronutrient focuses on one gender.

Disclaimer: This is not medical advice. Always talk to your healthcare providers (doctor, registered dietitian, pharmacist, etc.) before beginning a dietary supplement, especially important when you prepare for pregnancy.

Micronutrients to Consider for Fertility

When it comes to fertility, some micronutrients get more than their fifteen minutes of fame. Do they deserve the hope and money invested? This section takes a closer look.

Carotenoids

Carotenoids are a class of more than 750 naturally occurring pigments synthesized by plants, algae, and photosynthetic bacteria. These molecules supply the rich yellow, orange, and red colors of many plants.

Some carotenoids are converted by the body into vitamin A; this form of vitamin A is called provitamin A and is found in fruits, vegetables, and plant-based products. The other type of vitamin A comes preformed and is found in food from animal sources.

β-carotene, alpha-carotene and β-cryptoxanthin have provitamin A activity. Other carotenoids found in food, such as lycopene, lutein, and zeaxanthin, are not converted into vitamin A but have antioxidant properties.

Fruit and vegetables provide most of the carotenoids found in the human diet.

Women

β-carotene acts as a potential antioxidant in the oocyte, possibly improving oocyte quality and ovarian function, according to one study.[355]

Men

Several carotenoids have been studied in relation to sperm parameters. A cross-sectional study published in 2019 reported the effects of β-carotene, β-cryptoxanthin, and lutein:[356]

- **β-carotene** is the most common form of carotene in plants and has been shown to diminish oxidative stress. Intake of β-carotene has been inversely related to DNA fragmentation index (DFI). DNA integrity can be adversely affected when freezing sperm.

- **β-cryptoxanthin** intake had a positive association with sperm density.

- **Lutein** intake was related to higher total sperm count.

Another antioxidant in the carotenoid family, lycopene is seen to have high concentrations in the testes. Lycopene supplementation improved sperm parameters and oxidative stress biomarkers in a cohort of oligozoospermia infertile men.[357] An earlier study also showed that lycopene was linked with total motile sperm counts in a study with healthy young men.[358]

Food sources of carotenoids include:*

- Leafy green vegetables (kale, spinach, collard), orange and yellow vegetables (carrots, sweet potatoes, pumpkin and other squash)
- Tomatoes
- Red bell pepper
- Cantaloupe, mango
- Beef liver
- Fish oils
- Fortified foods

* The carotenoids discussed here (β-carotene, β-cryptoxanthin, lutein and lycopene) are available in varying amounts in the foods listed.

Carotenoid supplements

Vitamin A is available in dietary supplements, usually in the form of retinyl acetate or retinyl palmitate (preformed vitamin A), beta-carotene (provitamin A), or a combination of preformed and provitamin A. You will find that most multivitamin-mineral supplements contain vitamin A. Dietary supplements that contain only vitamin A are also available.

RDAs for vitamin A are given as retinol activity equivalents (RAE) to account for the different bioactivities of retinol and provitamin A carotenoids, all of which are converted by the body into retinol.

RDAs for Vitamin A range from 400 mcg retinol activity equivalents (RAE) for infants to 6 months on up to 1300 mcg for breastfeeding women.

High intakes of vitamin A can be harmful. There is a distinction in this regard between preformed vitamin A and provitamin A. Getting too much preformed vitamin A can cause dizziness, nausea, headaches, coma, and even death. High intakes of preformed vitamin A in pregnant women can also cause birth defects in their babies.

The daily upper limits for preformed vitamin A range from 600 mcg for babies to 12 months on up to 3000 mcg for adults 19 years and older.

Conversely, consuming high amounts of beta-carotene or other forms of provitamin A can turn the skin yellow-orange, but this condition is harmless (and so much safer than a tanning booth). High intakes of beta-carotene do not cause birth defects or other serious effects caused by getting too much preformed vitamin A. Upper limits for beta-carotene and other forms of provitamin A have not been established.

For more information, consult the NIH Office of Dietary Supplements Health Professional Fact Sheet on Vitamin A.[359]

VITAMIN C

Vitamin C, also known as L-ascorbic acid, is a powerful antioxidant and is involved in collagen synthesis and other protein metabolism. It improves the absorption of non-heme iron (not from meat), a mineral that grows in importance during pregnancy.

Unable to be made by the body, vitamin C must be obtained from the diet or supplements.

Women

Vitamin C deficiency is associated with an increased risk of preeclampsia. Some studies have shown that supplementation with multivitamins can lower the risk of preeclampsia in normal or underweight women.[360]

Men

Vitamin C improves the function of testicular enzymes and increases testosterone production. In sperm cells, vitamin C prevents agglutination and protects against DNA damage caused by ROS molecules.[361]

A clinical trial found that taking 1 gram of vitamin C for 2 months reduced the rate of sperm DNA fragmentation in the infertile men.[362]

Another trial, this time with obese men, revealed that consuming 1 gram of vitamin C as a supplement every other day improved sperm concentration and mobility.[363]

In couples undergoing ART, men's vitamin C intake was positively linked with fertilization rates in a 2019 study.[364]

Food sources of vitamin C include:

- Citrus fruit (oranges, kiwi, lemon, grapefruit)
- Bell peppers
- Strawberries
- Tomatoes
- Cruciferous vegetables (broccoli, Brussels sprouts, cabbage, cauliflower)
- White potatoes
- Fortified foods and beverages

Vitamin C supplements

Vitamin C is widely available in multivitamins and as single supplements, usually in the form of ascorbic acid but other forms are also acceptable.

RDAs begin at 40 mg for infants up to 6 months of age and reach 120 mg for breastfeeding women. Smokers are told to add 35 mg to their vitamin C intake to repair damage caused by free radicals. For infants under 1 year, breast milk and infant formula have adequate amounts of vitamin C but cow's milk does not.

People who get little or no vitamin C (below about 10 mg per day) for many weeks can develop scurvy, which can lead to anemia and even death.

Excess vitamin C intake can be harmful, leading to iron overload.

The daily upper limits for vitamin C are not established for babies up to 1 year of age. For children ages 1-3, 400 mg is recommended and 2000 mg for adults is the highest recommended amount.

For more information, refer to NIH Office of Dietary Supplements Health Professional Fact Sheet on Vitamin C.[365]

VITAMIN D

Vitamin D is a hormone produced naturally in the skin in the presence of the sun's ultraviolet rays. Deficiencies of the "sunshine vitamin" are common. As many as one billion people worldwide have low levels of vitamin D.[366]

Many people have limited sun exposure, especially during winter; dark skin individuals produce a type of melanin pigment that protects against ultraviolet ray damage but also reduces vitamin D synthesis.[367]

Others at risk include obese people and those with inflammatory bowel diseases, which disrupt normal fat digestion required for vitamin D metabolism.

Few foods contain vitamin D naturally. Fortified foods provide most of the Vitamin D in diets. People who do not eat milk, eggs, and fish (such as those with lactose intolerance or who follow a vegan diet) are at higher risk for a deficiency.

Vitamin D aids in both calcium and phosphorus absorption and metabolism, critical for building bone. The vitamin also reduces inflammation and modulates cell growth, glucose metabolism, and neuromuscular and immune function.

Vitamin D receptors and vitamin D metabolizing enzymes are also found in reproductive tissues of women and men leading to the suggestion of a role for vitamin D in fertility.[368]

In addition, vitamin D regulates the expression of endogenous antioxidant enzymes and deficiencies may cause reductions in glutathione, an important antioxidant.[369]

Quite a few studies have investigated vitamin D status relative to reproductive health.

Women

Women with vitamin D intake below estimated average requirements may be less likely to conceive.[370]

Vitamin D deficiency in pregnant women is associated with an increased risk of complications such as pre-eclampsia, bacterial vaginosis associated preterm delivery, gestational diabetes mellitus and small-for-gestational-age births.[371]

Vitamin D may have a role in endometrial receptivity and implantation based on a diverse cohort of 99 recipients that revealed lower pregnancy rates in vitamin D deficient recipients of egg donation.[372]

Women experiencing recurrent miscarriages showed higher rates of vitamin D deficiency in one study.[373]

In PCOS, low vitamin D levels are linked to obesity, metabolic disorders, and endocrine disturbances; bringing vitamin D levels back to normal may improve menstrual frequency and metabolic disturbances in these women.[374]

Ovarian reserve showed a positive correlation with vitamin D concentration among women over 40 years of age, in one study.[375]

But another study of 283 infertile women younger than 42 years old concluded that vitamin D deficiency had no detrimental effect on ovarian reserve.[376]

In patients undergoing ART, vitamin D deficiency had negative effects on egg and embryo quality, as well as on reproductive function.[377]

But vitamin D status did not affect pregnancy rates following the transfer of thawed frozen embryos,[378] or when implementing euploid embryo transfers.[379]

And finally, a meta-analysis reviewing data from 2,700 patients reported that the ART live birth rate was significantly higher in the vitamin D sufficient group than in both the insufficient group and deficient group. No significant difference in miscarriage rates was identified.[380]

Men

A key role for vitamin D in the male reproductive system is suggested, stemming from the observed expression of vitamin D receptors and metabolizing enzymes in the testis and spermatozoa.[381]

Vitamin D is positively associated with semen quality and androgen status. Moreover, vitamin D treatment may increase testosterone levels.[382]

However, in a 2020 review of the impact of vitamin D on male fertility, which looked at available animal and human models, the conclusions were anything but conclusive. The main findings were controversial for some seminal parameters, although they confirmed that vitamin D may have a positive effect on human male fertility potential. Notably, normal levels of vitamin D seem to be related to higher pregnancy rates. The authors of the review concluded, "Future studies are needed to better clarify the exact role of vitamin D on hormonal and seminal panel in both fertile and infertile men."[383]

Food sources of vitamin D include:

- Cod liver oil
- Fatty fish
- Mushrooms exposed to ultraviolet light
- Orange juice fortified with vitamin D
- Dairy and plant milks fortified with vitamin D

- Beef liver
- Egg yolk
- Fortified cereals

Vitamin D supplements

Due to widespread deficiencies caused by inadequate exposure to sunlight as well as insufficiencies in diet, supplements are often necessary.

The two forms of vitamin D in a variety of supplements are D2 (ergocalciferol) and D3 (cholecalciferol). Both forms increase vitamin D in your blood, but D3 may raise it higher and for longer than D2. Because vitamin D is fat-soluble, it is best absorbed when taken with a meal or snack that includes some fat.

The RDA per day ranges from 400 IU (10 mcg) for infants to 800 IU (20 mcg) for adults older than 70 years. Pregnant and lactating women are advised to get 600 IU (15 mcg).

Too much vitamin D can be harmful, almost always caused by consuming excessive amounts of vitamin D from dietary supplements. Very high levels of vitamin D in your blood (greater than 375 nmol/L or 150 ng/mL) can cause nausea, vomiting, muscle weakness, confusion, pain, loss of appetite, dehydration, kidney stones, and excessive urination and thirst. Extremely high levels of vitamin D can cause kidney failure, irregular heartbeat, and even death.

FYI: *Tolerable Upper Intake Level (UL): maximum daily intake unlikely to cause adverse health effects.*[384]

There are established daily upper limits for vitamin D including intakes from all sources—food, beverages, and supplements. These upper limits range from 25 mcg (1,000 IU) in newborns to 100 mcg (4,000 IU) for those over 9 years of age and also pregnant and lactating women.

For more specific information on vitamin D, refer to NIH Office of Dietary Supplements Health Professional Fact Sheet on Vitamin D.[385]

Vitamin E

Vitamin E is a fat-soluble antioxidant. In addition to protecting cells from the damage caused by free radicals, vitamin E is integral to the immune system and circulatory system. Deficiencies are rare in healthy people but a few studies found supplementation to be beneficial in reproduction.

Women

In women undergoing controlled ovarian stimulation, supplementation with vitamin E significantly increased endometrial thickness compared with no supplementation. Results were thought to be due to both antioxidant and anticoagulant effects.[386]

Men

Vitamin E serves multiple functions in male fertility, including biosynthesis of testosterone and modulation of telomerase activity.

Treatment of asthenospermic patients with oral vitamin E improved sperm motility in one study.[387] Earlier research also found improvement in sperm function.[388]

Most other studies paired vitamin E with other supplements making it difficult to tease out the impact of vitamin E alone.[389] For example, in one clinical trial, Vitamin E paired with selenium improved sperm quality and had beneficial effects on sperm motility in infertile men.[390]

Food sources of vitamin E include:

- Wheat germ oil
- Sunflower, safflower, and soybean oil
- Sunflower seeds
- Almonds
- Peanuts, peanut butter
- Green vegetables such as collard greens, spinach and broccoli
- Pumpkin
- Red bell pepper

- Mango
- Avocado
- Fortified foods

Vitamin E supplements

Vitamin E supplements come in different forms. Although vitamin E sounds like a single substance, it is actually the name of eight related compounds in food, including alpha-tocopherol. Each form has a different potency or level of activity in the body.

Vitamin E from natural sources is commonly listed as d-alpha-tocopherol on food packaging and supplement labels whereas synthetic vitamin E is listed as dl-alpha-tocopherol. The natural form is twice as potent: 1 mg d-alpha-tocopherol is equal to 2 mg dl-alpha-tocopherol.

If you come across a label listing vitamin E in International Units (IUs) rather than mg, use this conversion:

- 1 IU of the natural form of vitamin E is equivalent to 0.67 mg.
- 1 IU of the synthetic form of vitamin E is equivalent to 0.45 mg.

As stated, vitamin E deficiency, though rare in healthy people, can cause nerve and muscle damage as well as a weakened immune system.

RDAs range from 4 mg for infants up to 6 months on up to 19 mg for breastfeeding teens and women.

Vitamin E in the diet is not known to be excessive but if in supplement form, caution is advised. High doses of vitamin E may interfere with the blood's clotting ability and increase the risk of serious bleeding in the brain (known as hemorrhagic stroke).

For more information, refer to NIH Office of Dietary Supplements Health Professional Fact Sheet on Vitamin E.[391]

VITAMIN B6

Vitamin B_6 is a water-soluble vitamin that is naturally present in many foods, added to others, and available as a dietary supplement. Your body needs vitamin B_6 for more than 100 enzyme reactions involved in metabolism. Vitamin B_6 is also involved in brain development during pregnancy and infancy as well as in immune function. Although not considered a classic antioxidant compound, vitamin B_6 has been shown to have highly efficient antioxidant effects.[392]

Deficiencies are not common among healthy people. But kidney diseases, malabsorption syndromes, genetic diseases, autoimmune disorders, alcohol dependence, and some medications can lead to deficiencies over time.

Just a few studies address vitamin B_6 in fertility.

Women

Women who are infertile appear to have lower vitamin B_6 levels than fertile women, as reported in a systematic review.[393]

Men

Research pinpointing vitamin B_6 taken in isolation for fertility is scarce. A metabolically active form of vitamin B_6 is needed as a cofactor for the enzymes that allow selenium to be used from the dietary form. Given selenium's role in male fertility (addressed later), vitamin B_6 status should be known if fertility issues arise.

Food sources of vitamin B_6 include:

- Beef liver
- Tuna
- Salmon
- Fortified cereals
- Chickpeas
- Poultry
- Many fruits and vegetables, especially bananas, avocados, cantaloupe, and dark leafy greens.

Vitamin B_6 supplements

Vitamin B_6 is available in multivitamin supplements as well as separately, usually in the form of pyridoxine.

RDAs range from 0.1 mg for babies up to 6 months to 1.3 mg for adults to 2.0 mg for breastfeeding teens and women. Pregnant teens and women should get 1.9 mg.

Taking high levels of vitamin B_6 from supplements for a year or longer can cause severe nerve damage, leading people to lose control of their bodily movements. The symptoms usually end when supplements are discontinued. Other symptoms of too much vitamin B_6 include painful skin patches, nausea, heartburn, and extreme sensitivity to sunlight.

The daily upper limits for vitamin B_6, which include intakes from all sources—food, beverages, and supplements—are not established for babies up to one year of age. But upper limits range from 30 mg for children ages 1 to 3 on up to 100 mg for adults.

For more information, refer to NIH Office of Dietary Supplements Health Professional Fact Sheet on Vitamin B_6.[394]

Folate and Folic Acid

Folate and folic acid are both forms of vitamin B_9. Folate occurs naturally in foods. Folic acid is the synthetic form available in supplements and fortified foods. Vitamin B_9 is involved in the synthesis of proteins and nucleic acids. Also needed to produce healthy red blood cells, vitamin B_9 is needed during rapid growth periods, such as during pregnancy and fetal development.

Vitamin B_9 deficiency is linked to a higher risk of having a baby with serious birth abnormalities including spina bifida (spinal defect) or anencephaly (a brain defect). Neural tube defects happen in the first few weeks of pregnancy; often before a woman finds out she is pregnant. Adequate levels are important for egg quality, maturation, fertilization, and implantation.

Since 1992, public health agencies have urged that all women of reproductive age consume 400 mcg of folic acid each day, in addition to consuming food with folate from a varied diet, to help prevent some major birth defects in the baby's brain.[395] Despite its availability in many foods, folate can be difficult to consume in adequate amounts. Therefore, folic acid is added to foods such as enriched bread, pasta, rice, cereal, and corn masa flour. Check the nutrition label on food packaging. Taking a supplement with a higher dose than 400 mcg of folic acid each day is not necessarily better for preventing a neural tube defect but may be better for optimum reproductive health.

Women

Among 269 infertile women attending an IVF clinic, only 12% had red blood cell folate levels considered optimal to prevent neural tube defects.[396]

In a prospective cohort study of 3895 Danish women who were planning a pregnancy, increased fecundability was reported after the use of folic acid compared with non-use. The greatest increases were observed in women with irregular, short or long menstrual cycles.[397]

Higher intake of folic acid from supplements was associated with a reduced risk of spontaneous abortion (miscarriage) among 11,072 women in the Nurses' Health Study II who self-reported a pregnancy between 1992 and 2009.[398]

Some evidence on the effect of folic acid risk of miscarriage is conflicting; however, the few studies that have adjusted for confounding support a protective effect.[399]

Among 232 women seeking assisted reproductive technology treatment in one study, higher total folate and folic acid intake was associated with higher rates of implantation, clinical pregnancy, and live birth. Live birth rates were 20% higher among women in the highest quartile of supplemental intake (more than 800 mcg/day) than among women in the lowest quartile (less than 400 mcg/day).[400]

In a 2022 study, the folate and folic acid intake of 552 infertile women were assessed by food frequency questionnaires. Higher intake, particularly from supplements, was associated with modestly higher ovarian reserve as measured by antral follicle count (AFC) among women attending a fertility center.[401]

Men

A literature search revealed that folate has a role in spermatogenesis. Folate can act as an antioxidant counteracting reactive oxygen species (ROS).[402]

Low concentrations of folate in seminal plasma may be detrimental to sperm DNA stability, evinced from one data set that compared healthy men to men visiting a fertility center.[403]

A 2021 intervention trial reported positive results with folic acid supplementation. A randomized group of 162 infertile men received daily supplements containing 15 mg of folic acid or a placebo for 3 months. Though no changes in sperm characteristics were observed, a decrease in DNA fragmentation in the folic acid group was seen. Notably, there was a higher clinical pregnancy rate in the folic acid group compared to the placebo group. High-dose folic acid supplementation in men requiring in vitro fertilization (IVF)-intracytoplasmic sperm injection (ICSI) for male infertility improves outcomes.[404]

Food sources of folate include:

- Dark green leafy vegetables (turnip greens, spinach, romaine lettuce, asparagus, Brussels sprouts, broccoli)
- Beans
- Peanuts
- Sunflower seeds
- Fresh fruits, fruit juices
- Whole grains
- Liver
- Seafood
- Eggs

- Fortified foods and supplements; many foods naturally contain folate, but the form that is added to foods and supplements, folic acid, is better absorbed.

Folic acid supplements

Folic acid is available in multivitamins and prenatal vitamins. It is also offered in B-complex dietary supplements and supplements containing only folic acid.

Folic acid is the form of folate that is commonly used in fortified foods and supplements but methylfolate (5-methyl-THF) can also be used. RDAs are expressed as micrograms (mcg) of dietary folate equivalents (DFEs). The measure of DFE is used because your body absorbs more folic acid from fortified foods and dietary supplements than it absorbs from folate found naturally in foods. Compared to folate found in foods, you actually need less folic acid to get recommended amounts. For example, 240 mcg of folic acid and 400 mcg of folate are both equal to 400 mcg DFE.

RDAs range from 65 mcg DFE in newborns to 600 mcg DFE in pregnant teens and women.

Importantly, because half of all pregnancies may be unplanned, all women and teen girls who could become pregnant should consume 400 mcg of folic acid daily from supplements, fortified foods, or both in addition to the folate they get from following a healthy eating pattern.

Folate that is naturally present in food and beverages is not harmful. However, you should not consume folic acid in supplements or fortified foods and beverages in amounts above the upper limit, unless recommended by a healthcare provider. Consuming large amounts of folic acid supplements may hide or worsen a vitamin B_{12} deficiency, which can lead to permanent damage to the brain, spinal cord, and nerves. In addition, high doses of folic acid may increase the risk of colorectal cancer and possibly other cancers.

The daily upper limits for folate are not established for babies up to 12 months of age. The daily upper limits established range from 300 mcg for children 1 to 3 years of age to 1000 mcg for adults 19 years and older.

For more information, refer to NIH Office of Dietary Supplements Health Professional Fact Sheet on Folate.[405]

VITAMIN B12

Vitamin B_{12} or cobalamin is essential in red blood cell formation, cell metabolism, nerve function, and the production of DNA, the genetic material in all cells. It also appears to have antioxidant properties.[406]

Deficiencies are not uncommon. They are usually due to disease, aging, or consuming a restricted diet.

Women

Inadequate vitamin B_{12} levels have been reported in more than half of the 269 women attending an infertility clinic for IVF.[407]

An earlier study also made this connection between vitamin B_{12} deficiency and female subfertility. Early deficiency may lead to loss of the fetus while a more prolonged deficiency may affect fertility by causing changes in ovulation or development of the ovum or changes leading to defective implantation.[408]

Men

A 2017 review of studies found generally positive effects of vitamin B_{12} on semen quality. Better sperm count and motility as well as reduced DNA damage were the primary observations.[409]

A study done in rats showed vitamin B_{12} to be protective against cimetidine-induced androgenic failure and sperm quality damage. This popular anti-ulcer drug is just one of many common medications with negative effects on reproductive health.[410]

Food sources of vitamin B_{12} include:

- Fish, shellfish
- Liver
- Red meat
- Poultry
- Eggs
- Dairy products such as milk, cheese, and yogurt
- Fortified nutritional yeast

- Fortified breakfast cereals
- Enriched soy or rice milk

Plant foods have no vitamin B_{12} unless they are fortified, which makes supplementation advisable for vegans. In addition, some people poorly absorb vitamin B_{12} from food or on medications that can interfere with absorption.

Vitamin B_{12} supplements

Vitamin B_{12} is available in multivitamins, single supplements, sublingual form (dissolved under the tongue), nasal gel and as a shot. It is usually in a form called cyanocobalamin.

RDAs for vitamin B_{12} range from 0.4 mcg for babies to 6 months on up to 2.8 mcg for breastfeeding teens and women. Pregnant teens and women should get 2.6 mcg.

Some supplements offer doses of vitamin B_{12} that are much higher than recommended amounts, such as 500 mcg or 1,000 mcg, but your body absorbs only a small percentage of it. These doses are thought to be safe.

For more information, refer to NIH Office of Dietary Supplements Health Professional Fact Sheet on Vitamin B_{12}.[411]

Chromium

Chromium appears to bolster insulin action. Indeed, this trace mineral is often recommended to help control blood sugar levels in diabetics. Low levels of chromium are linked with gestational diabetes, a condition in which glucose blood levels are elevated during pregnancy in a woman not previously diabetic.

Women

After eight weeks of treatment, chromium supplementation in non-pregnant women with PCOS (an insulin-resistant condition) led to an increase in pregnancy rate.[412]

Another study found that eight weeks of chromium supplementation in infertile women with PCOS led to improvements in biomarkers of inflammation and glucose.[413]

Food sources of chromium include:

- Grape juice
- Brewer's yeast
- Orange juice
- Beef
- Turkey breast
- Tomato juice
- Apples

Chromium is present in many more foods but amounts vary depending on local soil and water conditions as well as processes used to produce them. Data on actual chromium intakes are limited. A healthy diet could very well supply enough but supplements may be suggested for improved blood sugar control and possibly fertility in some women.

Chromium supplements

Most multivitamin/mineral supplements contain chromium. Supplements containing only chromium are also available, and they commonly provide 200 mcg to 500 mcg of chromium, although some contain up to 1,000 mcg.

When evidence is insufficient to develop an RDA, an Adequate Intake (AI) level may be established. AIs for chromium range from 0.2 mcg for infants up to 6 months on up to 45 mcg for breastfeeding adult women.

Upper limits have not been established but caution is advised for those with kidney and liver disease. High amounts may also interfere with medications.

Dietary supplements contain many forms of chromium. Chromium picolinate is better absorbed than another common form called chromium chloride.

For more information on chromium, refer to NIH Office of Dietary Supplements Health Professional Fact Sheet on Chromium [414]

Other Micronutrients

The following micronutrients are known potent antioxidants along with acting in other key roles. The vitamins mentioned earlier may also provide antioxidant effects, as noted.

ZINC

As a trace mineral, zinc is needed only in small amounts. Yet its influence is vast, required by almost 100 enzymes in vital chemical reactions. In addition to its work in DNA formation, zinc has a major role in building proteins, healing damaged tissue, bolstering the immune system, and supporting rapid growth, as in pregnancy. Zinc has been studied relative to fertility in both women and men.

Women

In females, zinc plays a role in sexual development, ovulation and the menstrual cycle. Zinc has antioxidant properties that counteract reactive oxygen species (ROS). Oocyte maturation, ovulation, luteolysis and follicle atresia are all affected by ROS.[415]

As noted in one study, women with low levels of zinc tended to take a longer time to achieve pregnancy.[416]

A review of 51 papers involving over 15,000 women and their babies revealed a small but significant reduction in preterm birth with zinc supplementation.[417]

Men

Zinc is involved in testicular development, sperm maturation and testosterone synthesis.[418]

It also functions as an antibacterial agent in the male urea system.[419]

A 2016 meta-analysis of 20 studies including 2,600 infertile males and 867 normal controls concluded that the zinc level in the seminal plasma of infertile males was significantly lower than that of healthy males.[420]

In one study, low serum zinc concentration was correlated with a higher risk of asthenozoospermia.[421]

In another trial, zinc therapy improved sperm parameters in men with asthenozoospermia.[422]

One study from 2002 reported total normal sperm count increased after combined zinc sulfate and folic acid treatment in both subfertile and fertile men.[423]

An intervention from the same medical center conducted several years later showed that combined zinc sulfate and folic acid treatment resulted in increased sperm concentration in subfertile males, though the mechanisms were not clear.[424]

A 2017 meta-analysis of six studies concluded that folic acid plus zinc supplementation had a positive effect on sperm concentration in subfertile men.[425]

But conversely, among a general population of couples seeking infertility treatment, the use of folic acid and zinc supplementation by male partners, compared with placebo, did not significantly improve semen quality or couples' live birth rates.[426]

In spite of these findings, previous studies on folic acid and zinc show antioxidant effects on improving sperm parameters;

the synergistic behavior of antioxidants in male fertility requires more study.[427]

Zinc cannot be stored in the body therefore daily intake is crucial.

Food sources of zinc include:

- Shellfish, especially oysters
- Beef
- Poultry
- Pork
- Legumes
- Nuts, seeds
- Whole grains
- Fortified cereals

Zinc supplements

Zinc is present in almost all multivitamin/mineral dietary supplements and is also available alone or combined with calcium, magnesium or other ingredients.

Dietary supplements can have several different forms of zinc including zinc gluconate, zinc sulfate and zinc acetate. It is not clear whether one form is better than the others.

Diet supplies adequate zinc for most people but certain groups may require supplements: those with digestive disorders or a history of gastrointestinal surgery; vegetarians; older breastfed babies; alcoholics; sickle cell disease patients.

RDAs range from 2 mg for infants up to 6 months on up to 13 mg for breastfeeding teens.

Excessive zinc can cause immediate symptoms including nausea, vomiting, loss of appetite, stomach cramps, diarrhea, and headaches. Long-term excess can lead to low copper levels, lower immunity, and low levels of HDL cholesterol (the good kind). Use of nasal sprays and gels that contain zinc has been associated with the loss of the sense of smell, in some cases long-lasting or even permanently. Oral products containing zinc, such as cold lozenges appear to not have these safety concerns.

The daily upper limits for zinc range from 4 mg for infants up to 6 months of age to 40 mg for adults.

For more information on zinc, refer to NIH Office of Dietary Supplements Health Professional Fact Sheet on Zinc.[428]

Selenium

Selenium is a trace mineral with a wide-ranging influence on reproduction, thyroid gland function, and DNA production. As a component of selenoproteins and enzymes, selenium acts as an antioxidant to protect the body from damage caused by free radicals, inflammation and infection.

Selenium status in both women and men appears to be a factor in fertility, as the following studies show.

Women

Research in animals and humans shows that selenium and selenoproteins are essential for optimal reproduction in females, likely because of their roles in the regulation and modulation of antioxidant balance.

In a 2019 study, women who had lower selenium concentrations had a longer time to attain pregnancy.[429]

However, the effects of maternal dietary selenium supplementation on oxidative stress and fetal ovarian development and function are poorly understood.[430]

Selenium supplementation appears to be of benefit in deficient individuals but potentially harmful in those with excess concentrations.[431] Caution is advised.

Men

Selenium is essential for testosterone biosynthesis and the formation and development of normal spermatozoa. Testicular tissue contains large concentrations of selenium and is responsible for sperm quality and male fertility health. In many animals, selenium deficiency is linked with poor reproduction. Supplementation improves performance in mice, sheep and cattle.

Selenium status in the human male also appears to be important to fertility.

In fertile men, selenium seminal plasma concentration is higher. Greater levels are linked positively with sperm parameters including motility, concentration, total count and morphology, as reported in a recent review.[432]

Selenium supplementation in a group of subfertile men with low selenium status improved sperm motility and the chance of successful conception. There was a 56% positive response to treatment.[433]

One later study in 468 infertile men with idiopathic oligo-asthenoteratospermia who were randomized to receive 200 mcg for 6 months showed improved semen volume, total sperm count and concentration, and morphology. Selenium supplementation may also be beneficial in men through its improvement of sperm motility.[434]

A small study enlisted 20 patients with chronic autoimmune thyroiditis, a condition linked to low selenium status. After supplementation, they showed improved sperm quality and a lower percentage of spermatozoa with DNA fragmentation compared with pre-treatment values.[435]

High levels of selenium may be detrimental according to some research. Semen levels greater than or equal to 80 ng/ml were associated with a high abortion rate and signs of ovarian dysfunction in the partner.[436]

Though results are conflicting, a study with 42 healthy men showed that selenium supplementation at levels near or slightly exceeding the upper safe limit (400 μg/d) had no impairment effect on conventional sperm parameters or serum hormones. Testes appeared to be as well protected from selenium excess as they were from deficiency.[437]

Selenium is found in many foods but the amount can vary widely depending on the selenium content of the soil in which it is grown for plants or in the case of meat, the content of the foods eaten by animals.

Food sources of selenium include:

- Brazil nuts*
- Fish
- Beef
- Poultry
- Whole wheat bread
- Beans
- Fortified cereals

*Brazil nuts contain very high amounts of selenium (68–91 mcg per nut) and can exceed the upper limit if you eat too many.

Selenium supplements

Selenium is available in many multivitamin-mineral supplements and other dietary supplements. It can be present in several different forms, including selenomethionine and sodium selenate.

RDAs range from 15 mcg for infants to age 6 months on up to 70 mcg for breastfeeding teens and women.

People undergoing kidney dialysis, living with HIV or those who eat only local foods grown in soils that are low in selenium may not get enough selenium.

Though rare in developed countries, selenium deficiency is implicated in heart disease, certain types of arthritis and as noted here, infertility.

Excess selenium can cause numerous problems including nausea, diarrhea, skin rashes, irritability, metallic taste in the mouth, garlic breath, hair and nail abnormalities, discolored teeth and nervous system problems.

Extremely high intakes of selenium can cause severe problems, including difficulty breathing, tremors, kidney failure, heart attacks, and heart failure.

The daily upper limits for selenium range from 45 mcg for infants to 6 months of age on up to 400 mcg for adults.

For more information, refer to NIH Office of Dietary Supplements Health Professional Fact Sheet on Selenium.[438]

Coenzyme Q-10

Coenzyme Q-10 (CoQ_{10}) is produced naturally in your body. One of its chief functions is to help generate energy in your cells. CoQ_{10} is also an effective antioxidant that protects cell membranes and lipoproteins from oxidation. About half of the body's CoQ_{10} is obtained through diet and the remainder is synthesized via the cholesterol metabolic pathway.[439]

Women

As a key antioxidant, CoQ_{10} has been tested in infertile women undergoing ART. A 2020 meta-analysis looked at five eligible randomized-controlled trials (449 infertile women; 215 in the CoQ_{10} group and 234 in the placebo/no treatment group). Oral supplementation of CoQ_{10} increased clinical pregnancy rate when compared with placebo or no-treatment. Even women with poor ovarian response and PCOS showed significant differences. No difference between groups was observed regarding live birth or miscarriage rates compared with placebo or no-treatment in women with infertility undergoing ART.[440]

And a 2020 review reported that CoQ_{10} supplementation showed positive effects both in young women with low ovarian reserve and in older women.[441]

Men

CoQ_{10} acts as an antioxidant, preventing lipid peroxidation of sperm cell membranes.[442]

Present in human seminal fluid, CoQ_{10} concentrations show a direct correlation with some seminal parameters (count and motility). Alterations of CoQ10 content were also shown in conditions associated with male infertility, such as asthenozoospermia and varicocele.[443]

In a 2015 clinical study, the usage of CoQ_{10} as a protective entity against oxidative stress and DNA damage was reported.[444]

A meta-analysis was done looking at the effect of CoQ_{10} treatments on male infertility. Three trials were included with 149 men in the CoQ_{10} group and 147 men in a placebo group. Though pregnancy rates were not higher, sperm concentration and motility showed improvements with treatment.[445]

CoQ_{10} intake from food was not related to semen parameters among 211 male subfertile men seeking evaluation. The mean dietary intake of CoQ_{10} in this study was 10-fold lower than the supplemental dose used in clinical trials showing improved sperm motility. CoQ_{10} intake from food alone may be insufficient to optimize semen parameters.[446]

Food sources of coenzyme Q-10 include:

- Organ meats, such as kidney and liver
- Chicken
- Beef
- Pork
- Fatty fish, such as salmon, sardines and mackerel
- Soybean and canola oils
- Spinach
- Broccoli

- Soybeans
- Whole grains

Coenzyme Q10 supplements

CoQ_{10} is sold as a dietary supplement but no RDA or upper limits have been established for any age group. Mild side effects such as insomnia or digestive upsets may occur; no serious side effects of CoQ10 have been reported. However, CoQ10 may interact with the anticoagulant (blood thinner) warfarin and the diabetes drug insulin, and it may not be compatible with some types of cancer treatment.

For more information, refer to NIH National Center for Complementary and Integrative Health Information on Coenzyme Q10.[447]

CARNITINES

Derived from an amino acid, carnitine (L-carnitine, L-acetyl-carnitine and propionyl-L-carnitine) transports fatty acids into cells to be processed for energy. Carnitine has been studied extensively because it is important to energy production and is a well-tolerated and generally safe therapeutic agent.

Women

Plasma carnitine concentrations decline in the course of pregnancy, perhaps caused by reduced synthesis due to inadequate iron status.[448]

Hexanoylcarnitine, a metabolite of carnitine, was found in one study to be higher in the urine of women who had a spontaneous miscarriage as compared to women who had healthy births. Three other carnitine metabolites were lower in women who miscarried.

These changes in carnitine metabolite levels indicate defects in oxidation processes. Supplementation for pregnant women with threatened miscarriages may reduce the risk of spontaneous miscarriage.[449]

Men

Carnitine is abundant in the epididymis, a long, coiled tube that stores sperm and transports it from the testes. The high levels suggest a key role in sperm metabolism, providing energy for use by spermatozoa. L-carnitine and L-acetyl-carnitine also protect cell membranes and DNA against damage induced by free oxygen radicals.

Many controlled studies have supported a potential positive effect of therapy with L-carnitine and its acyl derivatives for male infertility.[450] A systematic review suggested that both versions of carnitines likely improve total sperm motility and reduce the percentage of sperm with atypical morphologies. In addition, the pregnancy rate was improved after the administration of carnitines in infertile men.[451]

Food sources of carnitine include:

- Red meat

- Fish
- Chicken
- Milk

Carnitine supplements

L-carnitine, acetyl-L-carnitine, and propionyl-L-carnitine are available as dietary supplements.

The body makes sufficient carnitine to meet the needs of most people. Dietary carnitine also contributes but mostly for people who eat red meat and animal products and not for vegans. The kidneys efficiently conserve carnitine, so even carnitine-poor diets have little impact on the body's total carnitine content.

Much research has explored the potential benefits of carnitine supplements in athletic performance, aging, Alzheimer's disease, cardiovascular disease, peripheral arterial disease, cancer treatment side-effect amelioration, type 2 diabetes, HIV and AIDS, as well as end-stage renal disease and hemodialysis. Notably, twenty years of research found no consistent evidence that carnitine supplements can improve exercise or physical performance in healthy subjects. Some research indicates that intestinal bacteria metabolize carnitine to form a substance called TMAO that may increase the risk of cardiovascular disease.[452] However, possible benefit is reported for the other conditions as well as male infertility.

No RDA or upper limits have been established for any age group. However, at doses of approximately 3 g/day, carnitine supplements can cause nausea, vomiting, abdominal cramps, diarrhea, and a "fishy" body odor. Rarer side effects include muscle weakness in uremic patients and seizures in those with seizure disorders.

For more information, refer to NIH Office of Dietary Supplements Health Professional Fact Sheet on Carnitine.[453]

MELATONIN

Melatonin is best known for its role in regulating the sleep-wake cycle. But this hormone has no snooze alarm. Many functions in the body hinge on the melatonin signal; these include antioxidant defenses and glucose regulation.[454]

Emerging evidence points to its significance in fertility.

Women

A 2020 review of 10 studies on women reported that melatonin treatment significantly increased the clinical pregnancy rate but not the live birth rate in ART cycles. Melatonin also improved the number of oocytes collected, maturated oocytes, and good quality embryos.[455]

Men

Compared to infertile men, fertile men were reported to have higher melatonin seminal and serum levels, both correlated to better sperm motility.[456]

Melatonin may reduce DNA fragmentation and improve sperm quality parameters in vitro.[457]

Many situations can disturb the complex nature of melatonin secretion. In one study example, workers on the night shift with extended light exposure showed diminished sperm concentration and motility as well as an increase of abnormal spermatozoa forms.[458]

A variety of foods provide melatonin, with huge variations noted.[459]

Food sources of melatonin include:

- Fruits such as tart cherries, cranberries, strawberries and grapes
- Fatty fish including salmon
- Nuts such as pistachios and walnuts
- Chicken
- Red meat
- Milk

Melatonin supplements

Melatonin dietary supplements can be made from animals or microorganisms, but they are most often made synthetically. Short-term use of melatonin supplements appears to be safe for most people, but information on the long-term safety of supplementing with melatonin is lacking. There's also a dearth of research on the safety of melatonin use in pregnant or breastfeeding women.

No RDA or upper limits have been established for any age group.

For more information, refer to NIH National Center for Complementary and Integrative Health Information on Melatonin.[460]

Inositol

Inositol is a promising antioxidant, but one with important distinctions depending on the type of stereoisomer (compounds differing only in the spatial arrangement of their atoms). Other beneficial effects include insulin-sensitizing properties, motility stimulation and hormonal regulation.

Myo-inositol (MI), the most abundant natural form of inositol, plays a pivotal role in reproductive physiology, while d-chiro–inositol (DCI) acts to a lesser extent. MI can be synthesized from D-glucose in the human body or can be derived from the diet or supplements.[461]

Women

MI plays a crucial role in oocyte and embryo development. The presence of MI sustains the progression of gestation.[462]

Both MI and DCI show potential for the treatment of insulin resistance and its associated metabolic and reproductive disorders, such as those occurring in women affected by PCOS. The combination of MI/DCI may be superior to either inositol species alone but the best ratio is not yet established.[463]

Ovarian function and response to ART improved when PCOS patients were given MI. A 2021 review reported that MI, at a dose of 4 g per day (2 g twice per day), three months before ovarian stimulation, was effective in normalizing ovarian function and improving oocyte and embryo quality in PCOS.[464]

Infertile non-PCOS patients undergoing ovulation induction for ICSI or IVF-ET also benefited when given MI. A review of 935 women from seven clinical trials showed more grade 1 embryos, improved pregnancy rate and reduced abortion rate. Also, a reduced amount of ovulation drugs was needed.[465]

MI and melatonin when supplemented together show a synergistic effect. In unassisted pregnancies, the combo enhanced gestational outcomes by contributing to embryo development. In IVF procedures, melatonin and MI, either administered to the patients or added to embryo culture media, showed an improvement in positive outcomes.[466]

Men

MI supplementation reportedly improved sperm quality and motility in patients with oligoasthenozoospermia (a sperm disorder that affects both sperm count and sperm motility) who are undergoing assisted reproduction techniques. Moreover, MI protected against oxidative damage to sperm DNA. On the other hand, DCI improves sperm quality by different mechanisms. A specific ratio of MI: DCI is crucial for the correct inositol-related functions.[467]

Inositols also play other roles. In addition to their antioxidant properties, the beneficial effects of inositols on sperm motility and mitochondrial function can be due to insulin-sensitizing properties, prokinetic activity and hormonal regulatory effects.[468]

Food sources of inositol include:

- Whole grains
- Fruits including prunes, cantaloupe, oranges, and grapefruit
- Beans
- Nuts including almonds and walnuts

Inositol supplements

Both forms of inositol, MI and DCI, are widely available in supplement form, alone or together. When combined, the usual ratio is 40:1 of MI to DCI though that proportion is not definitive.

A therapeutic dose of 4000 mg MI daily (2000 mg twice a day) is considered by some to be the best option for the improvement of metabolic alterations and prevention of gestational diabetes.[469]

No RDA or upper limits have been established for any age group. Inositol is defined as generally recognized as safe (GRAS) by the Food and Drug Administration (FDA).

In clinical trials in which MI dosages ranged from 4 to 60 g/day and the exposure time ranged from 1 to 12 months, the only adverse events reported were mild gastrointestinal symptoms (nausea, flatus, and diarrhea) and only at doses greater than 12 g per day.[470]

No side effects were observed in patients receiving intervention with DCI (27.5 up to 500 mg/day) in the available clinical studies.[471]

For more detailed information, refer to the above studies on inositol.

L-Arginine

L-arginine (also known as arginine) is an interesting amino acid because it is conditionally essential depending on the developmental stage and health status of the individual. For example, preterm infants are unable to create L-arginine internally, making the amino acid essential for them. But most healthy people can synthesize L-arginine from glutamine and glutamate via citrulline in the kidneys. In addition, L-arginine is plentiful in protein-containing foods.

In the body, L-arginine is converted into nitric oxide, a compound that dilates blood vessels, allowing better blood flow. L-arginine also stimulates the release of growth hormones, insulin and other substances in the body. Because of its vasodilation effects, L-arginine has been used for various conditions linked to circulatory problems: angina (chest pain), peripheral heart disease, erectile dysfunction and hypertension. It may lower blood pressure in healthy people, diabetics, people with pulmonary hypertension, and pregnant women with high blood pressure who may develop preeclampsia. L-arginine may also benefit infants with necrotizing enterocolitis (NEC).

Women

In a small study of nine women, L-arginine treatment of 6 g/daily improved blood flow in eight patients and endometrial thickness in six patients.[472]

Supplementation of L-arginine together with magnesium and salicylate in women with a high-risk pregnancy for chronic hypertension already treated with low dose aspirin showed a trend towards improvement in blood pressure values and a lower need for a new antihypertensive treatment.[473]

Men

L-arginine has been shown to improve sperm quality, probably by the generation of nitric oxide. [474]

A 2021 review looked at the few studies done on L-arginine supplements and sperm parameters. In one study, human semen with low sperm motility incubated with L-arginine showed enhanced motility. In addition, several clinical studies of men seeking assistance at fertility clinics found better sperm parameters with L-arginine treatment.[475]

Food sources of L-arginine include:

- Fish
- Red meat
- Poultry
- Soy products
- Whole grains
- Beans
- Milk

L-arginine supplements

L-arginine is available as an oral and topical supplement; it can also be given intravenously.

No RDA or upper limits have been established for any age group.

L-arginine is generally recognized as safe (GRAS).

Reported side effects include nausea, abdominal pain, diarrhea, bloating, gout, headache, allergic response and worsening of asthma symptoms.

In addition, people with recent heart attacks or a history of cold sores and genital herpes should abstain.

For more information, refer to NIH Office of Dietary Supplements Health Professionals Fact Sheet on Dietary Supplements for Exercise and Athletic Performance.[476]

N-ACETYL-CYSTEINE

N-acetylcysteine (NAC) displays effective antioxidant activity. NAC is widely available as a dietary supplement but is actually a prescription drug approved by the FDA (to treat liver side effects from an overdose of acetaminophen and to loosen thick mucus in the lungs of people with cystic fibrosis or chronic obstructive pulmonary disease). Notably, the FDA recently stated that NAC should be excluded from the definition of a dietary supplement.[477]

Women

In one study, a combination of NAC and folic acid compared with folic acid alone improved pregnancy outcomes in patients with unexplained recurrent pregnancy losses.[478]

In a large study of patients with PCOS, those treated with clomiphene citrate plus NAC versus clomiphene citrate alone showed an improved ovulation rate.[479]

Men

A review of several studies with various designs and outcomes* reports that NAC may enhance fertility by:[480]

- Improved sperm quality (motility, count and morphology)
- Reduced DNA fragmentation
- Increased testosterone levels
- Reduced reactive oxygen species in the serum and reduced viscosity of the semen

*Some outcomes were seen in individual studies only

N-acetyl-cysteine supplements

Despite recent FDA warnings, NAC supplements remain available.

No RDA or upper limits have been established for any age group.

Side effects can include nausea, vomiting, abdominal pain, diarrhea, indigestion, and heartburn.

For more information, refer to NIH Office of Dietary Supplements Health Professionals Fact Sheet on Dietary Supplements in the Time of COVID-19.[481]

Resveratrol

Resveratrol is an organic compound, produced by some plants in response to cutting or threats from pathogens. Favorable results in animal and limited human trials suggest resveratrol may be an effective phytochemical for reproductive health.

Animals

Resveratrol treatment produced striking results in a trial with a mouse model fed with resveratrol for 12 months.[482] The treated female mice:

- Retained the capacity to reproduce, while age-matched controls produced no pups.
- Exhibited a larger follicle pool.
- Telomerase activity, telomere length and age-related gene expression in ovaries of mice fed with resveratrol resembled those of young mice.
- Showed improved number and quality of oocytes.

In another study, resveratrol treatment reduced the size of adipocytes and improved estrus cyclicity in a rat model of polycystic ovary syndrome (PCOS).[483]

Humans may benefit too. Resveratrol acts as an effective antioxidant in addition to possessing cardioprotective, neuroprotective, anti-inflammatory and anticancer activities.[484]

Women

Mounting evidence suggests that resveratrol has potential therapeutic effects in infertile women who have diminished ovarian function, polycystic ovary syndrome (PCOS), or endometriosis.[485]

Ovarian function

Loss of oocytes and follicles and reduced oocyte quality contribute to age-associated ovarian aging and infertility. Follicle quality has been enhanced with low doses of resveratrol, possibly due to reduced oxidative stress in the ovarian environment.[486] Resveratrol also activates telomerase activity and mitochondrial function, improving ovarian function.[487]

PCOS

A clinical trial in women with PCOS found that resveratrol reduced ovarian and adrenal androgens, thought partly due to an improvement of insulin sensitivity and a decline in insulin level. However, the fertility outcome has not been evaluated.[488]

Endometriosis

In addition, resveratrol may exercise its anti-inflammatory properties in the prevention of endometriosis, a condition that can lead to infertility. A recent review of the epidemiological and clinical research supports the beneficial effect of resveratrol in endometriosis.[489]

In IVF, the addition of resveratrol to in vitro culture media may benefit human oocytes, leading to improved oocyte maturation and developmental competence of embryos.[490]

Adverse effects

Recall that during decidualization, the endometrium is made receptive for implantation and maintenance of pregnancy. An inflammatory reaction is needed for embryo implantation.

However, as an anti-inflammatory, resveratrol may suppress the required response. In a recent clinical study, patients in the resveratrol treatment group had poor pregnancy outcomes after IVF-embryo transfer (ET) cycles even though good quality embryos were transferred. Resveratrol intake was significantly associated with low clinical pregnancy rates and high miscarriage rates.[491]

Conversely, in a 2020 study, resveratrol supplementation was shown in vitro to enhance decidualization.[492] The discrepancies were thought to be due to the timing of the treatments to modulate the response during different phases of decidualization.[493]

Erring on the side of caution, treatment may hypothetically be used to improve oocyte quality but then stopped before decidualization so as not to impair implantation. A potential solution for infertility treatment may be to discontinue resveratrol (with a half-life of only 9-10 hours) at the beginning of the luteal phase (day of ovulation) or cryopreservation of embryos and pregnancy. [494] More clinical studies are needed to establish optimal doses and periods of resveratrol intake while preventing any adverse effects on implantation, subsequent pregnancy, and the fetus.

In conclusion, resveratrol treatment has been shown to protect against ovarian aging and improve PCOS and endometriosis; therefore, resveratrol intake may have benefits for some patients. But it also may have adverse effects on implantation and endometrial decidualization. As described above, resveratrol treatments may need to be carefully timed to respect these striking differences in effect.

Men

Freezing semen (cryopreservation) can damage sperm. The addition of resveratrol was shown to avoid oxidative damages post-thaw but did not restore the decrease in sperm motility.[495]

Environmental toxins and medications can be toxic to male reproduction. In rodent studies, resveratrol (RSV) had positive impacts against several toxins:

Polyvinyl chloride (synthetic plastic polymer): RSV reduced oxidative stress.[496]

Acrylamide (formed in some foods during cooking): RSV ameliorates the DNA damage in both germ cells and spermatozoa but long-term treatment caused premature activation of these cells.[497]

Valproic acid, a drug for epilepsy: RSV minimized drug damage and protected the male reproductive system.[498]

And finally, a disease state such as Type 1 diabetes mellitus can increase oxidative stress. RSV treatment improved the lipid peroxidation and DNA fragmentation seen in this disease, which is increasing in numbers.[499]

Food sources of resveratrol include:

- Wine (though best avoided by aspiring parents)
- Grapes, blueberries and cranberries

- Cocoa and dark chocolate
- Nuts such as peanuts and pistachios

Resveratrol supplements

No RDA or upper limits have been established for any age group.

Resveratrol supplements may contain anywhere from less than 1 mg to 1600 mg of resveratrol per tablet or capsule, but there isn't any specific dosage recommendation.

Adverse effects resulted mainly from long-term use (weeks or longer) and daily doses of 1000 mg or higher, causing nausea, stomach pain, flatulence, and diarrhea.[500]

Important: Supplementation should be discontinued during pregnancy, based on the adverse decidualization effects in the human endometrium.

For more information, refer to NIH MedlinePlus Information on Resveratrol.[501]

ALPHA-LIPOIC ACID

Alpha-lipoic acid (ALA) is a natural short-chain fatty acid and potent antioxidant.

Women

A 2021 review reported that ALA had positive effects on multiple processes from oocyte maturation to fertilization, embryo development and reproductive outcomes.[502]

Men

ALA oral supplementation has been shown to improve sperm quality parameters.[503] ALA also appears to reduce DNA fragmentation in both thawed[504] and non-frozen sperm.[505]

In addition, short-term treatment with ALA along with glutathione in dyspermic men at two fertility clinics improved the reproductive outcomes of the IVF procedure.[506]

Food sources of alpha-lipoic acid include:

- Organ meats including beef liver
- Vegetables including spinach, broccoli, tomatoes, peas and Brussels sprouts

Alpha-lipoic acid supplements

No RDA or upper limits have been established for any age group.

Used as a dietary supplement, alpha-lipoic acid has been demonstrated to be safe in 610 expectant mothers who had been treated daily by oral route with 600 mg alpha-lipoic acid, for at least 7 weeks during gestation. No adverse effect was noticed in mothers or newborns.[507]

Possible adverse effects are being further monitored in ongoing studies.

For more information, refer to this NCBI Resource on Alpha-Lipoic Acid.[508]

ANTIOXIDANT THERAPY FOR FERTILITY

An early review assessed the impact of antioxidant supplements on infertile men. Nineteen of the 20 studies showed a significant reduction relating to some measure of oxidative stress in human spermatozoa.[509]

A 2018 review of 26 studies reported a positive effect of antioxidant therapy on basic semen parameters, advanced sperm function, outcomes of assisted reproductive therapy, and live-birth rate.[510]

And in another 2018 review, the authors recommended that antioxidant supplements should be encouraged, especially in men undergoing infertility treatment, although the specific antioxidants and doses remained unclear.[511]

A systematic review of the available clinical evidence was performed in 2021. Based on 97 studies, a significant number showed the beneficial effects of oral antioxidants in improving semen parameters and pregnancy outcomes. Antioxidant treatment in specific clinical conditions, including varicocele, unexplained and idiopathic male infertility, and cases of altered semen quality, also looked promising. However, the researchers pinpointed factors that hinder their acceptance and use in male infertility: lack of randomized placebo-controlled studies that show the safety and efficacy of antioxidants in improving pregnancy rates in infertile couples in addition to a lack of consensus on the type of antioxidant to be used, dose, duration of treatment, and costs. The available evidence on antioxidant supplements in the clinical conditions involved in male infertility can be viewed in a Table available online from this review.[512]

A 2021 study tasked 77 men who had had low fertilization rates in their previous intracytoplasmic sperm injection (ICSI) cycles to take an antioxidant mix of myo-inositol, alpha-lipoic acid, folic acid, coenzyme Q10, zinc, selenium, and vitamins B_2, B_6, and B_{12}. After 90 days of treatment, sperm quality and concentration improved from baseline. Fertilization, embryo quality, and blastocyst development were significantly higher after treatment.[513]

Antioxidant treatment may be warranted if the condition is caused by oxidative stress. Unfortunately, specific antioxidants and dosages remain unclear. Monitoring is recommended to avoid over-dosage and to establish success.

Thoughts on Supplements

In a perfect world, a healthy diet would be consumed by everyone. Unfortunately, that is far from reality. Social, economic, educational, ethnic, cultural, and genetic factors can intervene, leaving many men and women of reproductive age lacking vital micronutrients. Moreover, we have imperfect knowledge of what an optimum diet even looks like, though we are getting closer.

Micronutrients have critical roles in fertility. Inadequate levels can impair the ability to conceive. Though data is not conclusive, supplementing with vitamins and minerals before conception for both healthy individuals and those struggling to conceive may enhance nutritional status and boost fertility.

Women

Female reproduction depends on micronutrients including antioxidants to function in an ideal manner.

According to the authors of a 2019 paper titled The Impact of Preconceptional Multiple-Micronutrient Supplementation on Female Fertility:

"Micronutrient supplementation can enhance the reproductive environment by helping restore micronutrients to recommended levels and strengthening the antioxidant defense system, thus ameliorating oxidative stress, with the clinical benefits of improving oocyte and embryo quality, reducing the time to conception, and increasing the chances of becoming pregnant."[514]

Women are introduced to micronutrient supplements at their first prenatal visit. Supplements containing folate (B_9) along with vitamins A, B_1, B_2, B_3, B_6, B_{12}, C, D and E as well as the minerals calcium, iron and zinc are often recommended. When infertility is an issue, supplements of a different order—newly researched antioxidants—may be advised.

Here, too, as with supplements for men seeking optimum fertility, it is important to stress the relatively unregulated nature of the supplement market for female fertility.

Men

As extensively described here, male fertility is highly dependent on optimum micronutrient status. Much research shows that oxidative stress plays a big part in the pathophysiology of male infertility and that antioxidants have a role in the treatment of male infertility.[515]

A look at the current marketplace reveals countless products to bolster fertility for men. And of course, these formulas are always changing as new research supports various micronutrients and doses for fertility.

For example, one study showed that consuming vitamin complements (30 mg of Q10, 8 mg of zinc, 100 mg of vitamin C, 12 mg of vitamin E, 400 mg of folic acid) once a day along with 200 mg of selenium every other day improved sperm parameters in infertile male smokers.[516]

Synergy

One plus one is not always two. Antioxidants may interact to make a combined effect greater than the sum of their separate effects—a dynamic called synergy.

For instance, melatonin and myo-inositol showed a synergistic effect in improving outcomes in unassisted pregnancies as well as in IVF procedures.[517]

Cautions on supplements

Caution #1: Popping a pill is easy. Much easier than planning, shopping, cooking, and consuming a healthful diet. But isolating nutrients involves many unknowns such as the differences between foods and supplements in absorption and metabolism. Many of the processes are not fully understood, making things such as bioavailability difficult to discern.[518]

People should get most of their nutrients from food and beverages, according to the USDA. In some cases, fortified foods and dietary supplements are useful when it is not possible otherwise to meet needs for one or more nutrients (e.g., during specific life stages such as pregnancy). For more information about building a healthy dietary pattern, see the Dietary Guidelines for Americans [519] and the U.S. Department of Agriculture's MyPlate.[520]

Caution #2: Most supplements are not controlled by strict regulation, as is true for food and drugs. A prescription is not needed to buy them in most countries. Supplements can be countless formulations, containing both nutrients and botanicals at different doses, and are readily available online as well as in brick and mortar stores. Moreover, information regarding recommendations for daily doses as well as upper limits to prevent toxicity is different in different countries. This book includes data from the United States only. Readers from other countries will want to consult a local health care expert regarding supplement types and dosage.

Disturbingly, because of a lack of stringent regulation, some supplements may not contain what is listed on the product label. For example, in a 2017 study, researchers tested 31 different melatonin supplements bought from grocery stores and pharmacies. Melatonin content did not come within a 10% margin of the label claim in more than 71% of supplements. Also, 26 percent of these supplements contained serotonin, a hormone that can have harmful effects even at relatively low levels.[521]

The FDA doesn't verify that supplements' content matches the labels nor does it check for contamination from heavy metals, bacteria, or pesticides. Some independent groups have taken on the role. In their December 2019 issue, Consumer Reports (a time-honored nonprofit consumer organization) summarized: "These groups include ConsumerLab.com, National Sanitation Foundation (NSF) International, and U.S. Pharmacopeia (USP). USP is a nonprofit organization that sets what Consumer Reports experts say are the most widely accepted standards for supplements. (It also sets mandatory standards for pharmaceuticals.) The not-for-profit NSF offers two types of certification: NSF Contents Certified and NSF Certified for Sport. ConsumerLab.com, a for-profit company, regularly tests and certifies supplements."[522] Cost to the manufacturer ranges from $3000 to $15,000+ per product tested. Given the investment, a manufacturer using these services is demonstrating a dedication to quality. Supplements with these designations may more reliably match content to label.

Caution #3: Indiscriminate use can be harmful. In the case of antioxidants, large doses may counteract the desired effect, a phenomenon called the "antioxidant paradox." Overuse of antioxidants such as selenium, vitamin C, vitamin E, and N-acetyl cysteine may lead to reductive stress, which is reported to be as dangerous to cells as oxidative stress. For example, selenium in seminal plasma at a higher than optimal range is associated with reduced sperm motility and elevated miscarriage rates.[523]

A 2020 systematic review of 21 dietary supplements available in Italy to improve sperm parameters reported interesting data:[524]

- Zinc was the most common ingredient (70% of products), followed by selenium, L-arginine, coenzyme Q, and folic acid. As reviewed before, these particular ingredients have evidence to vouch for benefits in fertility.
- The majority contained a large number of ingredients, up to 17, which could lead to issues such as low amounts of each substance and a high risk of interactions.
- Nutrients were often present at a dosage below minimal effective daily dose.

- Supplements frequently exceeded the safe upper limits for some nutrients while others had sub-optimal dosages.
- Some ingredients included had no scientific evidence of efficacy (i.e., astragalus, vitamin D_3, taurine and riboflavin).
- Added plant extracts may interact with drug metabolism.

Caution #4: Many if not most of these micronutrients in supplement form can interact with medications and other supplements. It is imperative to tell your doctor, pharmacist, and other healthcare providers about any dietary supplements and medicines you take. They should be able to tell you if your supplements could interact or interfere with your prescription or over-the-counter medicines or conversely if the medicines might interfere with how your body uses nutrients. You can also research interactions at Dietary Supplement Fact Sheets (nih.gov).[525]

Final words on supplements

Given the observed shortcomings and possible harms, supplements should be carefully scrutinized for composition and dose that will address a patient's personal needs.

Supplements, as with most nutrients, pose a goldilocks scenario. Often a U-shaped curve shows harm at both ends of the spectrum. Too much or too little can damage health.

Aim for the sweet spot in supplement use. Consult a dietitian or doctor with knowledge of optimum levels of intake. A personalized approach is best.

Part Six: Putting It All Together

Genetic evolution drives the marriage of egg and sperm on a glorious journey to shape new life. The ride is not easy. All along the way, the elegant and complex physiological processes—many still unexplained—can be derailed by unfavorable conditions. The best example of this may be how chromosomal abnormalities can lead to miscarriage, as if some wiser force is protecting the child from a grim future. But many other damaging factors may disrupt fertility, implantation, fetal growth and safe birth. A child's health may also suffer, even into adulthood.

These harmful influences have multiplied in the 21st century. Modern life with all its stress, anxieties, unhealthy food, pollution, and workplace demands is not conducive to creating new life. Our bodies push back, making infertility, miscarriages and problem pregnancies more likely. Nonetheless, identifying the source of such obstacles to healthy reproduction can point you to better lifestyle choices.

Wherever you are on the quest to have a child, it is crucial to prepare as best as possible by following the latest evidence about enhancing fertility. Reducing stress and chemical exposures are obvious first steps.

Stress causes both physical and emotional changes that can impact fertility. Research shows links to lower sperm quality in men and higher rates of miscarriage in women. Stress must be—and indeed can be—managed. Meditation, moderate exercise, a healthy diet, and probiotics are all effective in managing stress and anxiety. Tobacco, alcohol, marijuana, anti-depressants and other commonly used balms are poor remedies for stress and may be part of the fertility problem. Seek help in quitting if you have a dependency.

More nuanced are the many ways our microbes, weight, diet and micronutrients can impact fertility and pregnancy. In this review, I have plumbed the latest research in hopes of adding guidance for healthy outcomes. Initially, I sought evidence linking these impacts on fertility. But it became quickly apparent that the entire journey, from conception to birth and beyond, is inextricably affected by microbes, diet, weight and micronutrients. The lifestyle choices you make before conception and up to delivery may predict failure or success.

Whether you are trying to conceive for the first time or are seeking professional help after a year or even years of attempts, the evidence is clear. Microbes matter. Weight matters. Diet matters. Micronutrients matter.

What's more, both men and women should heed the message. Both partners are responsible for creating a healthy baby.

By condensing the extensive research covered earlier, the following sections highlight the key concepts as well as steps you can take to enhance fertility and increase your odds for a healthy pregnancy and child. This section may be used as a stand-alone guide for patients and practitioners or for those less inclined to delve into the science behind the recommendations.

Also, note that this summary includes endnotes or hyperlinks for new references only. Sources for all of the supporting evidence can be accessed in the corresponding sections or the bibliography.

MICROBES

The microbiome is a new frontier in reproductive health. The past few decades of research give strong evidence that your microbes—both women's and men's—are important actors. This is welcome news. It adds another target—one which may be easier (and far cheaper) to address—for couples preparing and/or struggling to conceive.

Women

Reproductive microbiota in healthy women of procreative age show low diversity (unlike healthy profiles seen in other regions such as the gut). Only a few lactobacilli species account for up to 95% of total bacteria.

Lactobacillus crispatus, *Lactobacillus gasseri*, *Lactobacillus iners*, and *Lactobacillus jensenii* are the most represented in the vagina of healthy women. Yet different women host different microbes, a distinction most apparent in Hispanic and Black women. Infertile women host a different microbiota than healthy and fertile women.

Lactobacilli and related organisms help maintain a healthy vaginal microbiota free of pathogens by several mechanisms: lactic acid, hydrogen peroxide, and bacteriocins production; physical barrier strengthening; immune activation.

Several common disorders may interfere with this ideal female reproductive system. Bacterial vaginosis (BV), endometriosis, pelvic inflammatory disease (PID) and polycystic ovary syndrome (PCOS) are all linked to poor reproductive outcomes. Dysbiosis (fewer lactobacilli and higher diversity) may lead to or result from inflammation and infections.

Antibiotics are the go-to treatment for infections. But in bacterial vaginosis (BV), for example, nearly half of women treated have a recurrence within one-year post-treatment. After all, antibiotics also kill the good pathogen-fighting microbes.

A better strategy may be to use probiotics alone (success has been seen in BV) or after the course of antibiotics to restore a healthy microbiota. Oral probiotics are the norm but vaginal application is faster and more targeted.

Several oral and vaginal probiotics containing *Lactobacillus* spp. are available in the marketplace. Many of them may include one or more of these species: *L. crispatus*, *L. gasseri*, *L. plantarum*, *L. reuteri*, and *L. rhamnosus*.

In regard to ART, success rates are improved when women have healthy low-diversity dominance with lactobacilli.

Colonizing the transfer-catheter tip with *Lactobacillus crispatus* at the time of embryo transfer may increase the rates of implantation and live birth rate while decreasing the rate of infection.

Taking Care of Vaginal Microbes

- Use only mild soaps and never douche.*
- Manage vaginal pH: a more acidic environment facilitates the growth of *Lactobacillus* species and inhibits pathogens.
- Include fermented foods and beverages at every meal if possible. Yogurt, kombucha, kefir, kimchi and fermented cheeses are the most known but other foods can be fermented too. The actual probiotic content is not established.
- Include prebiotic foods so that your beneficial microbes can flourish. Plants that are rich in prebiotics include onions, garlic, bananas, chicory root, and Jerusalem artichokes. Prebiotics added to foods or supplements include galacto- oligosaccharides (GOS), fructo-oligosaccharides (FOS), oligofructose (OF), chicory fiber, and inulin.
- Eat a healthful diet such as the Mediterranean diet.
- Avoid tobacco and alcohol.
- Exercise regularly.

- Consider a supplement (with probiotic bacteria described before) that may repopulate the bacteria known to exist in a healthy ecosystem.

* The term, douche, which means "to wash" or "to shower" in French, is often done with prepackaged products. The solution can alter the normal pH as well as the balance of bacteria in the vagina. Though commonly practiced (among Black women especially) and touted in ads targeting women, vaginal douching is linked to many adverse outcomes including BV, cervical infection, PID, ectopic pregnancy (implantation of a fertilized egg outside the uterine cavity), cervical cancer and as a risk factor for HIV acquisition.[526] The American College of Obstetricians and Gynecologists (ACOG) recommends that women avoid vaginal douching.[527]

Men

Semen delivers sperm but also vital nutrients for a successful pregnancy. Once thought to be a sign of infection, bacteria in semen are now known to compose a microbiome, which can impact the fertilization and growth of a healthy fetus.

A man's seminal microbiota can be healthy or unhealthy. Ensuring a healthy seminal microbiome is an important step in health measures before trying to conceive. And know that making sure your microbiota is in good shape is recommended for all men—not just the infertile—who wish to optimize the health of their future child.

Certain strains of lactobacilli may have a protective role in the male genital tract, similar to what is seen in females.

If pathogens (e.g. *Escherichia coli, Chlamydia trachomatis*) prevail and lactobacilli are reduced, sperm function and quality will suffer. Pathogens drive inflammation and oxidative stress ensues, a condition that is linked to infertility, reduced sperm motility, sperm DNA damage and increased risk of recurrent abortions and genetic diseases. Some 30% to 80% of male sub-fertility may be associated with oxidative stress that damages spermatozoa and can decrease the success of in vitro fertilization (IVF) techniques.

Though antibiotics have traditionally treated these pathogens, increasing antibiotic drug resistance calls for alternate therapies. Correcting dysbiosis of the microbiota to deter pathogens is a solution with big potential.

Probiotics

Probiotics are thought to enhance male fertility through improved sperm parameters and testosterone levels. Several studies using selected strains of lactobacilli in animals and humans showed positive effects.

Prebiotics too were able to ameliorate some semen parameters in both animal models and humans.

Combining the two in a synbiotic may be even better in improving sperm parameters and improving testosterone levels.

Actions:

- Include fermented foods and beverages at every meal if possible. Yogurt, kombucha, kefir, kimchi and fermented cheeses are the most known but other foods can be fermented too. The actual probiotic content may be variable.
- Include prebiotic foods so that your beneficial microbes can flourish. Plants that are rich in prebiotics include onions, garlic, bananas, chicory root, and Jerusalem artichokes. Prebiotics added to foods or supplements include galacto- oligosaccharides (GOS), fructo-oligosaccharides (FOS), oligofructose (OF), chicory fiber, and inulin.
- Consider a supplement (with probiotic bacteria described before) that may repopulate the bacteria known to exist in a healthy ecosystem.

Couples Therapy

Partners share microbes during sexual intercourse. This "seminovaginal" microbiome may foster harmful or helpful exchanges of organisms.

Takeaway

Probiotics may boost fertility in both men and women. Altering the microbiome has been shown to enhance male fertility by reducing oxidative stress and improving testosterone levels and sperm quality. And in women, probiotics may restore a healthy genital tract with predominant *Lactobacillus* species, preventing pathogens from upending the balance, which can lead to complications, such as bacterial vaginosis, pre-term birth in pregnancy, and infertility.

In 2010, I launched www.ProbioticsNow.com[528] to share the cascade of new discoveries regarding the microbiome. Always amazed at this "forgotten organ," I also create white papers, blogs, videos and social media for the International Probiotics Association[529] as well as continuing education platforms. Tap into these resources for all things probiotic and to keep current with the latest information on the microbiome and reproductive health.

Weight

As stated before, obesity rates in the United States have reached a staggering 40% in both women and men between 20 and 39 years, putting a large swath at health risk in their prime reproductive years. The causes are many—not only excess calories or poor self-control—as I wrote about in *Globesity: 10 Things You Didn't Know Were Making You Fat.*[*530] My 2013 book delves into the science linking pollution, crime, drugs and seven other suspects to the obesity pandemic. Unhappily, updates must report that the problem has only gotten worse. Obesity rates keep rising. And seemingly in tandem, fertility is dropping. If we keep this up, the human species may be in trouble.

On my website, ProbioticsNow.com, [531] you can access a few chapters of the book at no cost. Better yet, enter your email for a chance to win a free book.

Overweight women

Obese women may face multiple challenges on the way to being a parent.

First, simply getting pregnant is more difficult. Obesity can impede fertility by contributing to anovulation (no release of an egg), irregular menstrual periods, adverse oocyte quality, endometrial alterations, and hormonal imbalances.

And then if pregnancy does occur, complications may include hypertensive disorders, gestational diabetes, preterm birth, and higher rates of cesarean delivery.

Moreover, obese women have less success with in vitro fertilization.

Though the existing data is scant and inconsistent, weight loss in obese women may help fertility and live birth rates. Weight loss programs using lifestyle modification in obese women have been shown to restore menstrual cyclicity and ovulation as well as improve the likelihood of conception. On the other hand, a recent trial in obese infertile women (a lifestyle intervention preceding infertility treatment compared with prompt infertility treatment) did not result in higher rates of vaginal birth in the treated women.

The lifestyle changes that are recommended to achieve weight loss—healthy diet and exercise—are without a doubt, even without weight loss, beneficial for reproductive, maternal pregnancy, and birth outcomes.

More women are choosing bariatric surgery to lose excess weight. In addition to generating swift and extreme weight loss, the procedure does appear to improve the polycystic ovary syndrome phenotype common in women with morbid obesity. Concerning however is an increased risk of small-for-gestational-age infants and a trend toward a higher risk of stillbirth and neonatal death with no reduction in preterm births, as seen in one study.

Increasing exercise or starting a regular program may support weight loss. But independent of weight reduction, physical activity in obese women undergoing fertility treatments has been shown in one study to increase pregnancies and live birth rates, tripling the chances compared to sedentary women.

All obese women should adopt healthy lifestyle changes before planning a pregnancy.

Underweight women

Women who are underweight and have low amounts of body fat may experience ovarian dysfunction and infertility. Preterm birth and/or low birth weight infants are also more likely.

Common reasons for being underweight include disease, drug use and energy deficiency. The last is seen in some athletes. A particularly thorny cause, which usually strikes young women in their reproductive years, is anorexia nervosa (AN). (Other eating disorders like bulimia and binge eating are more apt to lead to overweight or obesity, which are also problematic).

Despite having a high rate of menstrual irregularities, women with AN are becoming pregnant. A history of AN that is under control may not reduce fertility as was once thought.

More good news: One review reported that past or recent AN does not appear to cause increased complications with most aspects of delivery.

But both recent and past AN can affect fetal well-being, manifested in some offspring as lower birthweights than in the general population. What's more, the long-term physical and mental health of the child may be endangered. Undernutrition and overexposure to stress hormones are the main processes that underlie negative fetal programming. These are also the core features of AN.

When preparing to conceive, women who are underweight—for whatever reason—should take steps to gain weight by eating a nutrient-dense diet as well as moderating excessive exercise. Extreme exercise can interfere with hormone levels and ovulation. Stress should be addressed through behavioral therapy, meditation and other lifestyle changes.

Overweight men

Obesity in men should not be discounted; it appears to be every bit as damaging to fertility and embryo health as in women.

Several studies have noted obesity as a factor in the decline in overall sperm quantity and quality in the last several decades.

Though contradictions were evident, obesity was observed to negatively affect several factors predicting male fertility: the testosterone to estrogen (T/E) ratio, ejaculate volume, sperm concentration, morphology, and total motile count.

When a couple seeks help via ART, outcomes seem to be different when the male is obese. The odds of conceiving can be lower and loss of pregnancy occurs more often.

Weight loss appears to improve semen parameters, with the largest weight loss showing the best results. One mechanism may be through the restoration of metabolic health, closely linked to sperm function.

All obese men should adopt healthy lifestyle changes before planning a pregnancy.

Underweight men

Being underweight can also impact male reproduction. One recent review observed that being underweight was linked to low sperm normal morphology.

A healthy body weight is important for increasing sperm quality parameters and potentially male fertility.

Takeaway

Being either overweight or underweight may harm fertility and reproduction, in both women and men. Once again, a U-shaped curve depicts harm at both ends of the weight spectrum. Consult a dietitian or fitness professional. Make a plan. Though it's never easy to begin, successful weight management depends on creating new habits. These beneficial changes can become just as sticky as harmful practices. Before you know it, you have adopted a healthy lifestyle: a walk in the woods becomes more enticing than a videogame on the couch, and fresh mango tastes better than greasy fries.

It takes some effort, but the rewards are great.

Diet

A healthy diet can make men and women more fertile.

Not surprising news perhaps, given the decades of research revealing the astonishing power of nutrition in the prevention and treatment of a long list of diseases and disorders.

Yet many people choose to ignore the facts. They regularly consume sugary beverages, fast foods and processed foods as their main food groups, what is embarrassingly dubbed the "Western diet." Tasty, cheap, and easy is a losing trifecta that has won over modern societies.

Laden with unhealthy fats and sugars that replace essential nutritious foods and beverages, the regimen can seriously harm fertility, pregnancy and offspring. The good news? Diet offers a valuable target for improving reproductive health because just about everyone has room for tweaks. But some may need dramatic changes in eating habits to enhance their fertility potential.

Women

As reported in this book, an impressive trove of data on diet and its impact on fertility is available through the Nurses' Health Studies. A "fertility" diet pattern (fewer trans fats and animal proteins and more low-glycemic carbohydrates, low-fat dairy, and multivitamins) was linked with a lower risk of ovulatory disorder infertility. Strikingly, it has been suggested that the majority of infertility cases due to ovulation disorders may be preventable through modifications to diet and lifestyle.

Similar in content, the Mediterranean Diet (fish and poultry, fruits, vegetables, whole grains and olive oil with limited red meat and dairy products) also begets fertility benefits. In one study, among non-obese infertile women under 35 years who consumed a Mediterranean Diet, the live birth rate was 20% higher than among those using other diet types.

The Pro-Fertility Diet is characterized by increased intake of whole grains, soy, seafood, dairy, low pesticide residue produce, and supplemental folic acid, B_{12}, and vitamin D. This more targeted approach may be appropriate for infertile women.

Men

In addition to the Mediterranean diet, several healthy dietary patterns, as well as the use of tools to measure adherence to recommended dietary guidelines, may benefit male fertility. Healthy Eating Index, Dietary Approaches to Stop

Hypertension, Alternate Mediterranean Diet Score and Alternative Healthy Eating Index are all linked with better sperm quality.

First and foremost, science shows that you must jettison the Western diet: red and processed meat, full-fat dairy products, refined grains, and sweets. If bacon, hamburgers, pizza, fries, chips, ice cream, and soda are your go-to menu items, it's best to rethink your choices. Plenty of healthful substitutions are tasty too. Grilled salmon, baked sweet potatoes, cinnamon applesauce, fresh greens, whole-grain rolls and sparkling water supply much-needed fiber, omega-3 fatty acids, antioxidants, vitamins, minerals and much more.

It is clear: the Western diet is linked with impaired reproductive function while healthful diets improve it.

Drilling down on what are called macronutrients (proteins, carbohydrates and fats), research provides some guidance on links to fertility and reproductive health.

Protein

Much research confirms that the source of protein is important for both men and women. Healthy protein sources are beans, nuts, low-fat dairy, fish, and poultry. Red meat and processed meat are not. Vegan, gluten-free and Paleo diets—to name a few popular regimens—can upend ordinary patterns of protein intake, frequently among young people of childbearing ages. Those adhering to such plans should seek help with ensuring suitable protein amounts and sources.

Carbohydrates

Cookies, cakes and potato chips are carbohydrates but are frequently manufactured from unhealthy simple sugars and starches packed with saturated fats. Instead, whole grain breads, grains, fruits and vegetables supply needed nutrients and fiber to your body. Several studies link the type of carbohydrate with fertility in both men and women.

Fats

Not all fats are created equal.

The amount and type of fat impact fertility and pregnancy, as well as sperm parameters.

Saturated fats and trans fats should be avoided. Embrace unsaturated fats of both monounsaturated and polyunsaturated types with a special focus on omega-3 fatty acids. But remember that total fat should also be limited. See the section on fats for details, as fats are markedly diverse.

Fatty processed meats are particularly harmful. Avoid hot dogs, sausage, bacon, beef jerky and cold cuts. For most people, full-fat dairy foods should be replaced with skim milk or low-fat products. Conflicting evidence on high-fat versus low-fat dairy benefits for women should spur more research.

For more information about building a healthy dietary pattern, see the Dietary Guidelines for Americans [532] and the U.S. Department of Agriculture's MyPlate.[533]

Takeaway

A healthy diet is nutrient-dense. Menus rich in fruits, non-starchy vegetables, nuts, legumes, seafood, vegetable oils, low-fat dairy, and whole grains with fewer red meats, processed (often sodium-preserved) meats, and foods high in refined carbohydrates and salt promote fertility and optimum pregnancy outcomes. To a dietitian such as myself, who has trumpeted good nutrition for a lifetime, the prescription seems simple enough. Keep your eye on the prize (a baby!) and ignore perverse food marketing, cheap deals, and lazy eating habits.

The Dietary Guidelines for Americans 2020-2025 recommend nutrient-dense forms of foods and beverages across all food groups, in recommended amounts, and within calorie limits.

MICRONUTRIENTS

They may not provide caloric energy like proteins, fats and carbohydrates, but micronutrients punch way above their weight across the spectrum of health.

As detailed before, vitamins, minerals and other micronutrients are needed in adequate amounts to prevent many serious problems like spina bifida. Micronutrient status affects fertility and reproduction processes all the way to a healthy birth and beyond.

The micronutrients singled out here are the ones identified as key players by the virtue of emerging evidence. Many are powerful antioxidants, sweeping up excess free radicals, which can damage cells and DNA. An imbalance, called oxidative stress, can imperil the best-laid parenting plans of mice (lab heroes) and men. And, of course, women. Fertility, pregnancy and delivery can be endangered.

Reducing oxidative stress in both men and women is paramount when planning a pregnancy. Fortunately, you can play a big part in this goal by changing your lifestyle and diet.

A healthy diet can supply most but not all micronutrients to optimize fertility and pregnancy. For more information about building a healthy dietary pattern (beyond what is included in this book), see the Dietary Guidelines for Americans and the U.S. Department of Agriculture's MyPlate. Consult a registered dietitian for personalized help.

Unfortunately, genetic and environmental factors can sabotage even the best of intentions. Poor choices are all too common today when fast food and processed goods dominate the landscape. Many women and men of reproductive age suffer from a suboptimal micronutrient status.

In some cases, fortified foods and dietary supplements are useful when it is not possible otherwise to meet needs for one or more nutrients. Here, I will briefly summarize the specific micronutrients that have evidence suggesting a role in reproductive health.

There are probably more, many more. Mysteries still abound. But research is unraveling how vital micronutrient nutrition is to that journey.

For each of the following, refer to the relevant section on micronutrients for more detailed information. There you will find the current evidence for use. Ranges of Recommended Dietary Allowances (RDAs) and upper limits of safe consumption, if available, are documented. Food sources and supplement information are also included.

The United States National Institutes of Health (NIH) Office of Dietary Supplements provides comprehensive information on most of these supplements including their roles in our health, metabolic activity, deficiencies, toxicities, recommended intakes, upper limits, interaction with medications and further reading. When available, the information I have included here is from this source. At times, research is reported for one gender only because that has been the focus for that particular antioxidant.

Disclaimer: this is not medical advice. Always talk to your healthcare providers (doctor, registered dietitian, pharmacist, etc.) before beginning a dietary supplement, especially important now when you prepare for pregnancy.

Carotenoids

Women: β-carotene acts as a potential antioxidant in the oocyte, possibly improving oocyte quality and ovarian function.

Men: As precursors of vitamin A, β-carotene and β-cryptoxanthin are linked to positive sperm parameters. Other carotenoids found in food, such as lycopene and lutein, are not converted into vitamin A but do improve sperm parameters and reduce oxidative stress.

Most multivitamins contain vitamin A. High intakes of preformed vitamin A (retinyl acetate or retinyl palmitate) can cause birth defects. Eat leafy greens and colorful vegetables.

Vitamin C

Women: Deficiency is linked with an increased risk of preeclampsia.

Men: Vitamin C may increase testosterone production, prevent sperm clumping and protect against DNA damage.

Many fruits and vegetables provide ample vitamin C. Supplementation in infertile men may improve outcomes.

Vitamin D

Women: Deficiencies have been linked to infertility, menstrual irregularities, miscarriages, pregnancy complications (such as pre-eclampsia, preterm delivery, gestational diabetes mellitus, and small-for-gestational-age births) as well as lower pregnancy and live birth rates in ART.

Men: Vitamin D sufficiency may have a positive association with semen quality and testosterone levels, though the research is conflicting.

Fortified foods and supplements are routinely used because few foods contain vitamin D naturally. Even if you spend much time in a sunny climate (producing vitamin D in your skin), you may be wise to supplement given its links to reproductive health.

Vitamin E

Women: The endometrium thickened with vitamin E supplementation in women undergoing ovarian stimulation.

Men: Vitamin E serves multiple functions in male fertility, including biosynthesis of testosterone and modulation of telomerase activity. Supplementation improved sperm parameters in asthenospermic patients.

Vitamin E in the diet is not known to be excessive but in supplement form, caution is advised because it may interfere with the blood's clotting ability.

Vitamin B_6

Women: Deficiencies have been linked to infertility.

Men: Research pinpointing vitamin B_6 in isolation for fertility is scarce.

Vitamin B_6 is widely available in foods and is usually included in multivitamins.

Folate

Women: Folate deficiency is linked to a higher risk of having a baby with birth defects including spina bifida or anencephaly.

Neural tube defects happen in the first few weeks of pregnancy; often before a woman finds out she is pregnant. Adequate folate levels are important for egg quality, maturation, fertilization, and implantation. ART outcomes may also benefit.

Men: Folate has a role in spermatogenesis. Supplementation in infertile men improved outcomes.

All women of reproductive age should consume a folic acid supplement in addition to consuming food with folate from a varied diet. Men may also benefit.

Vitamin B_{12}

Women: Deficiencies have been linked to infertility.

Men: Deficiencies have been linked to infertility and supplementation shows positive effects on semen quality.

Plant foods have no vitamin B_{12} unless they are fortified, which makes supplementation especially advisable for vegans.

Chromium

Low chromium levels are linked with gestational diabetes.

Women: Women with PCOS (an insulin-resistant condition) showed an increase in fertility after chromium supplementation. Another study revealed improvements in biomarkers of inflammation and glucose control with chromium supplements.

Though many foods provide chromium, supplements may be beneficial for some women.

Zinc

Women: Zinc plays a role in sexual development, ovulation and the menstrual cycle. Low levels were associated with a longer time to achieve pregnancy. A small but significant reduction in preterm birth was seen with zinc supplementation.

Men: Zinc is involved in testicular development, sperm maturation and testosterone synthesis. The zinc level in the seminal plasma of infertile males was significantly lower than in healthy males. Supplements improved sperm parameters in men with asthenozoospermia. Zinc may act together with folate to improve sperm parameters.

Diet supplies adequate zinc for most people but certain groups may require supplements.

Selenium

Women: Selenium and selenoproteins are essential for optimal reproduction, likely through antioxidant actions.

Men: Selenium is essential for testosterone biosynthesis and the formation and development of normal spermatozoa. Supplementation in infertile men improved sperm quality and reduced DNA damage.

Selenium is found in many foods. Supplements in excess amounts can be harmful as with some foods, especially Brazil nuts.

Coenzyme Q-10

CoQ_{10} is promising for its role in rescuing oxidative stress-induced damages.

Women: Supplements in infertile women showed an increase in clinical pregnancy rate even in women with PCOS and poor ovarian response.

Men: CoQ_{10} concentrations show a direct correlation with healthy sperm parameters.

Many foods contain CoQ_{10} but supplements may be needed to optimize antioxidant benefits.

Carnitines

Derived from an amino acid, carnitine (L-carnitine, L-acetyl-carnitine and propionyl-L-carnitine) transports fatty acids into cells to be processed for energy. Carnitine has been studied extensively because it is important to energy production and is a well-tolerated and generally safe therapeutic agent.

Women: Carnitine metabolite levels (both low and high) are linked to miscarriage indicating defects in energy production.

Men: Carnitines provide energy for sperm metabolism and protect against free oxygen radicals. They likely improve sperm quality and may improve the pregnancy rate when used by infertile men.

Our bodies make sufficient carnitine and the kidneys conserve it, meeting the needs of most people. Supplements may not be necessary.

Melatonin

Many functions depend on this hormone including immunity, antioxidant defenses, and glucose regulation.

Women: Melatonin treatment significantly increased the clinical pregnancy rate but not the live birth rate with infertile women using ART.

***Men*:** Melatonin may reduce DNA fragmentation and improve sperm quality parameters. Workers on the night shift with extended light exposure showed diminished sperm parameters.

A variety of foods provide melatonin, with huge variations noted. Supplementation of melatonin could be another option.

Inositol

Women: Myo-inositol (MI), the most abundant natural form of inositol, plays a crucial role in oocyte and embryo development. Supplements improved ovarian function and embryo quality in PCOS patients seeking ART. Non-PCOS patients also showed better quality embryos as well as improved pregnancy rate and reduced abortion rate. Women with both unassisted and assisted pregnancies benefited when given MI and melatonin together.

Men: MI treatment improved sperm parameters and protected against oxidative damage to sperm DNA in patients with sperm disorders who used ART. Another form called d-chiro–inositol (DCI) improves sperm quality by alternate mechanisms.

Also available in food, both forms of inositol, MI and DCI, are widely available in supplement form, alone or together. When combined the usual ratio is 40:1 of MI to DCI though that is not clearly established.

L-arginine

In the body, L-arginine is converted into nitric oxide, a compound that dilates blood vessels allowing better blood flow. L-arginine has been used for various conditions linked to circulatory problems.

Women: L-arginine treatment has shown improved blood flow and endometrial thickness in some women.

Men: L-arginine has been shown to improve sperm parameters in infertile men.

Widely available in food, L-arginine supplements may be helpful for those who need to lower blood pressure.

N-acetyl-cysteine (NAC)

Women: N-acetylcysteine (NAC) improved pregnancy outcomes when combined with folate.

Men: NAC may increase sperm quality and testosterone levels as well as reduce DNA fragmentation.

Used primarily as a prescription drug to treat cystic fibrosis, chronic obstructive pulmonary disease and acetaminophen overdose, NAC is available as a dietary supplement. But the FDA recently stated that NAC should be excluded from the definition of a dietary supplement.

Resveratrol

Women: Resveratrol treatment may protect against ovarian aging and have positive effects in PCOS and endometriosis. But supplementation has been strongly linked with a decrease in clinical pregnancy rate and an increased risk of miscarriage during fresh or frozen embryo transfer cycles. One solution for infertility treatment may be to discontinue resveratrol (it has a half-life of only 9-10 hours) during the luteal phase and pregnancy.

***Men*:** Freezing semen or cryopreservation can damage sperm. The addition of resveratrol was shown to evade oxidative damages post-thaw but did not restore the decrease in sperm motility. Resveratrol has also shown positive effects against environmental toxins and medications that can be toxic to male reproductive function.

As wine is not advised for hopeful parents, best to enjoy the many other delicious sources. Be cautious with supplements.

Alpha-lipoic acid (ALA)

Women: This short-chain fatty acid may have positive effects on oocyte maturation, fertilization, embryo development and reproductive outcomes.

Men: ALA may improve sperm quality parameters and reduce DNA fragmentation in both thawed and non-frozen sperm.

Organ meats and various vegetables provide ALA. Supplement recommendations are unresolved.

Takeaway

Clearly, both women and men benefit from addressing micronutrient deficiencies.

Supplementation in women can restore micronutrients to recommended levels (if such guidelines are available) and reduce oxidative stress, thereby optimizing fertility and reproduction.

Women are prescribed micronutrient supplements at their first prenatal visit. Supplements containing folic acid (B_9) along with vitamins A, B_1, B_2, B_3, B_6, B_{12}, C, D and E as well as the minerals calcium, iron and zinc are often recommended. When infertility is a concern, additional supplements such as newly researched antioxidants may be in order.

Men don't have prenatal visits. But the evidence gathered here suggests it would be a wise move. Male fertility is highly dependent on optimum micronutrient status. Much research shows that oxidative stress plays a big part in the origins of male infertility. Many studies show the beneficial effects of supplementary antioxidants in improving semen parameters and pregnancy outcomes.

As detailed in the *Thoughts on Supplements* section, supplements must be viewed with the utmost caution, especially by men and women planning pregnancy. Supplements may not be the best substitute for a healthy diet. They are not strictly regulated and large doses can be harmful and even interact with medications and other supplements.

Supplements, as with many nutrients, can show harm at both ends of the intake spectrum. Too much or too little can damage health. Take the utmost care when choosing supplements.

Consult a dietitian or doctor with knowledge of optimum levels of intake.

Final Thoughts

Creating a baby is art and science. The magic happens with a brilliant choreography of reproductive systems.

Preparing for a dance of a lifetime—and the health of your children and grandchildren and so on—may require a few or even many changes. Basic lifestyle choices must be examined. This is true whether you are trying to conceive for the first time or are seeking professional help after a year of attempts. Avoiding alcohol, tobacco, drugs, stress and environmental toxins is mandatory. Exercise moderately. Optimize your microbiota. Aim for a healthy weight. Consume nutrient-dense foods. Supplement when necessary.

If you are starting from a position of many bad habits, the needed changes may seem daunting. But it also means you have a long runway with many possible targets and hence potentially much reward. Nobody's perfect. Know that bad habits when challenged will become good habits, and just as durable.

Both fertility and your future child depend on your lifestyle choices today.

Personalized approach for fertility

Of course, you are unique.

What works for one person may not for another.

Diets, probiotics and supplements are not one-size-fits-all remedies, as the legions of special diets and preferences attest. For example, how does a gluten-free diet fit into all this? What if you follow a strict vegan or perhaps a FODMAP diet? Or one of the other modified diet plans designed for the 21st century?

A personalized approach is best.

My website ProbioticsNow.com brings you all the latest research on the microbiome. Science is always evolving. The COVID-19 pandemic best illustrates how scientific data can change from one study to the next. That's how science works. Debate, discussion and consensus building lead to the truth. Believe in the science and you will be prepared to benefit from its findings. In the case of fertility, all the recommendations gathered in this book on microbes, weight, and nutrition may lead to your goal: a baby.

Whether you are just starting on the quest to parenthood or have been trying for a long time, you want the absolute best for your future child.

Start now. A life depends on you.

Glossary

Acrosome reaction: The release of enzymes when a sperm encounters the protective coating of the egg allowing fusion with the plasma membrane of the egg.

Adipocyte: A specialized cell of adipose tissue (also called a fat cell) that stores excess energy in the form of triglyceride droplets and secretes various substances (such as leptin) that play a role in various physiological processes (such as regulation of food intake or lipid metabolism).

Adipokines: Bioactive molecules released by adipose tissue that interact with numerous metabolic pathways including oocyte differentiation and maturation. For example, altered levels of an adipokine such as leptin can disturb the developing embryo.

Agglutination: Clumping of sperm cells due to antigen-antibody reactions or infection.

Amenorrhea: The complete absence of menstrual periods.

Amniocentesis: At about 16 weeks of pregnancy, a small amount of amniotic fluid is removed through a needle from the fetal sac and then analyzed for chromosomal abnormalities.

Anencephaly: A serious birth defect in which a baby is born without parts of the brain and skull.

Aneuploidy: Having one or a few chromosomes above or below the normal chromosome number.

Angiogenesis: Growth of new blood vessels.

Antibiotic: A substance able to inhibit or kill bacteria.

Antral follicle count: The number of fluid-filled follicles detected using ultrasound.

Apoptosis: Programmed cell death.

Aspermia: Lack of semen

Assisted reproductive technology (ART): Medical procedures used primarily to address infertility; may include procedures such as in vitro fertilization, intracytoplasmic sperm injection, cryopreservation of gametes or embryos, and/or the use of fertility medication.

Asthenozoospermia: Reduced motility of sperm.

Atresia: In relation to the ovaries, the natural process by which eggs age and degenerate.

Azoospermia: Condition in which there is no measurable sperm in a man's semen caused by a lack of production or blockage.

Bacterial vaginosis: Vaginal inflammation caused by the overgrowth of bacteria that upsets the natural balance.

Bacteriocins: Proteins produced by bacteria that inhibit or kill the growth of other kinds of bacteria.

Bariatric surgery: Surgery on the stomach and/or intestines to help a person with extreme obesity lose weight.

Biofilm: A thin and usually resistant layer of microorganisms that form on and coat various surfaces.

Blastocyte: A thin-walled hollow structure in early embryonic development that contains a cluster of cells.

Cervical os: The internal os of the cervix is the opening of the cervix that joins the uterus. The external os of the cervix is the junction between the cervix and the vagina.

Corpus luteum: Hormone-secreting structure formed in an ovary at the site of a follicle or sac that has matured and released its ovum (egg) in the process known as ovulation.

Cytokines: Proteins that are crucial in controlling the growth and activity of other immune system cells and blood cells.

Decidualization: Dramatic changes in the cells of the endometrium in preparation for pregnancy.

DNA fragmentation: A change in one or both of the DNA strands of the chromosomes contained within the sperm.

Donor egg: An egg from a fertile woman that is donated to an infertile woman to be used in an assisted reproductive technology procedure.

Donor sperm: Sperm donated by a fertile man who is not the recipient's partner.

Dysbiosis: An imbalance in the microbial community associated with disease due to the gain or loss of microbes or changes in their relative abundance.

Embryo: Earliest stage of development after sperm fertilizes an egg.

Endometriosis: Disease where tissue similar to the lining of the uterus grows outside the uterus.

Endometrium: The layer of the uterus in which the implantation of the fertilized egg takes place. If the implantation does not occur, the functional (outermost) layer of the endometrium is shed and expulsed, leading to menstruation.

Epithelial cells: The inner lining of the vagina consisting of multiple layers of cells. The number of cell layers varies during the days of the estrous cycle, increasing from 22 layers on Day 10 to 46 on Day 14, when the glycogen level in the cells is at its highest immediately before ovulation. The vaginal epithelium helps prevent pathogenic microorganisms from entering the body by generating a mucous layer in which immune cells reside and by making antimicrobial peptides.

Estradiol: The predominant estrogen produced by the follicular cells of the ovary.

Estrogens: Female sex hormones produced by the ovaries responsible for the development of female sex characteristics and thickening of the uterine lining in preparation for ovulation and possible pregnancy.

Eumenorrhea: Normal menstrual bleeding which lasts 3-7 days and occurs every 21-45 days.

Fecundity: The physiological maximum potential reproductive output of an individual (usually female) over its lifetime.

Fertility: Current reproductive performance of an individual.

Fertilization: The fusion of sperm and egg.

Follicle atresia: The degeneration and resorption of several follicles and their ovules prior to the maturation and release of one ovule from a healthy follicle.

Follicle: A fluid-filled sac containing an egg and cells that produce hormones.

Follicle-stimulating hormone (FSH): A hormone made in the pituitary gland integral to reproduction in both men and women. In females, it acts on the ovaries to make the follicles and eggs grow. In males, it acts on the testes to produce sperm.

Genetic: Refers to genes, the basic units of biological heredity, which are contained on the chromosomes, and contain chemical instructions that direct the development and functioning of an individual.

Gestational Diabetes: A condition characterized by an elevated level of glucose in the blood during pregnancy, typically resolving after birth.

Glycemic Index: A number from 0 to 100 assigned to a food, with pure glucose arbitrarily given the value of 100, which represents the relative rise in the blood glucose level two hours after consuming that food.

Glycemic Load: A number that accounts for how much carbohydrate is in a food and how much each gram of carbohydrate raises blood glucose levels. Glycemic load is calculated by multiplying the grams of available carbohydrate in the food by the food's glycemic index and then dividing by 100.

Gonadotropin: Hormone that is secreted by the pituitary gland and affects the function of the male or female gonads.

Gonads: A reproductive gland such as an ovary or testis that produces germ cells (gametes).

Hormone: A substance secreted from organs of the body, such as the pituitary gland, adrenal gland, or ovaries, which is carried by a bodily fluid such as blood to other organs or tissues where it exerts a specific action.

Human Microbiome Project: Multiple projects undertaken across the globe, which seek to design strategies to manipulate our microbiota so as to optimize its performance in the context of an individual's physiology.

Hypospermia: Semen volume below normal.

Hypothalamic-pituitary-ovarian (HPO) axis: A tightly regulated system controlling female reproduction.

Hypothalamus: A thumb-sized area in the brain that controls many functions of the body, regulates the pituitary gland, and releases a gonadotropin-releasing hormone.

Idiopathic sperm abnormalities: When the cause of infertility is unknown as is the case in up to 30% of infertile men.

Immunomodulation: Modification of the immune response or the functioning of the immune system caused by agents that activate or suppress its function.

In vitro fertilization (IVF): A method of assisted reproduction that combines an egg with sperm in a laboratory dish. If cell division results in an embryo, it is transferred to the uterus. IVF is often the treatment for women who have damaged or absent Fallopian tubes.

Infertility: Inability to become pregnant after one year (or longer) of unprotected sex.

Insemination: Sperm is placed via syringe into a female's uterus or cervix to produce a pregnancy.

Intracytoplasmic Sperm Injection (ICSI): A tiny needle is used to inject a single sperm into the center of the egg. Once fertilization occurs, the fertilized egg (now called an embryo) grows in a laboratory for 1 to 5 days before it is transferred to the woman's uterus (womb).

Lactic acid or lactate: A byproduct of anaerobic respiration, the process by which cells produce energy without oxygen. In this context, lactic acid is a byproduct of lactobacilli metabolism and contributes to an acidic environment or lower pH.

Luteinizing hormone (LH): Hormone produced by the pituitary gland that, in the female, stimulates maturation of the ovarian follicle and formation of the corpus luteum, and in the male, the development of tissue in the testis.

Luteolysis: Structural demise of the corpus luteum, which is preceded by loss of the capacity to synthesize and secrete progesterone.

Mediterranean Diet: Fish and poultry, plentiful fruits, vegetables, whole grains and olive oil with limited red meat and dairy products compose this diet. One study showed that the live birth rate among non-obese women under 35 years, those following a Mediterranean diet was 20% higher than among those using other dietary approaches.

Menopause: The time of life when a woman's ovaries stop producing eggs and estrogen levels decline. Natural menopause usually occurs around age 50 but can be sooner or later. A woman is said to be in menopause when she hasn't had a period for 12 months in a row.

Menses: Menstrual periods, which are normal vaginal bleeding that occurs as part of a woman's monthly cycle. Every month, a woman's body prepares for pregnancy. If no pregnancy occurs, the uterus, or womb, sheds its lining.

Metabolic endotoxemia: Diet-induced increase in plasma liposaccharide levels which drives inflammation leading to the development of disease.

Metformin: A hypoglycemic drug that potentiates the action of insulin; used in the treatment of type 2 diabetes mellitus.

Microbiome: The collective genomes of bacteria, viruses, bacteriophages, protozoa, and fungi that symbiotically inhabit the human body.

Miscarriage: The spontaneous loss of a pregnancy before the 20th week.

Monounsaturated fats (MUFAs): A type of unsaturated fat with only one (mono) double bond, found in high concentrations in olive, peanut, and canola oils, avocados, nuts and seeds.

Nurses' Health Studies: Originated in 1976, the first cohort followed 121,700 married women through biannual surveys. The astonishing 90% response rate by these nurses over decades contributed greatly to public health. The studies have expanded through the years with additional cohorts.

Oligoasthenoteratozoospermia: A condition that includes oligozoospermia (low number of sperm), asthenozoospermia (poor sperm movement), and teratozoospermia (abnormal sperm shape).

Oligoasthenozoospermia: Combination of asthenozoospermia (reduced sperm motility) and oligozoospermia (low number of sperm).

Oligospermia: A low sperm count defined as lower than normal if you have fewer than 15 million sperm per milliliter of semen.

Oocytes or ova: Also called eggs, the germ cells produced by the ovaries that, when fertilized by a male's sperm, produce embryos.

Ovarian reserve: A woman's fertility potential. Diminished ovarian reserve is seen with depletion in the number of eggs and deterioration of oocyte quality.

Ovaries: The two female sex glands, one on each side of the uterus. The ovaries produce eggs and hormones including estrogen, progesterone, and androgens.

Ovulation: A follicle releases a mature egg on approximately the 14th day of a 28-day menstrual cycle.

Oxidative stress: An imbalance between the systemic manifestation of reactive oxygen species and a biological system's ability to readily detoxify the reactive intermediates or to repair the resulting damage.

Pelvic inflammatory disease (PID): An infection in the upper reproductive organs, such as the uterus, fallopian tubes or ovaries.

Pituitary gland: A pea-sized endocrine gland just beneath the hypothalamus in the brain that controls the ovaries, thyroid, and adrenal glands through the secretion of hormones.

Disorders may lead to irregular or absent ovulation in the female and abnormal sperm production in the male.

Polycystic Ovary Syndrome (PCOS): A condition marked by irregular periods, excess androgen hormone and polycystic ovaries (fluid-filled sacs surround the eggs).

Polyunsaturated fats (PUFA): So-called healthy fats, these long-chain carbon compounds, especially fatty acids, have two or more double bonds between the carbon atoms. PUFAs are found in high concentrations in sunflower, corn, soybean, and flaxseed oils, walnuts, flax seeds, cold-water fish and canola oil.

Prebiotic: A substrate that is selectively utilized by host microorganisms conferring a health benefit.

Preeclampsia: A serious condition of late pregnancy characterized by a sudden rise in blood pressure, edema, and leakage of large amounts of the protein albumin into the urine.

Preterm birth: When a baby is born too early, before 37 weeks of pregnancy have been completed.

Probiotics: Live microorganisms that, when administered in adequate amounts, confer a health benefit on the host.

Pro-Fertility Diet: Characterized by increased intake of whole grains, soy, seafood, dairy, low pesticide residue produce, and supplemental folic acid, B_{12}, and vitamin D.

Progesterone: Female hormone secreted by the corpus luteum in the ovary during the second half of the menstrual cycle that prepares the lining of the uterus for implantation of a fertilized egg.

Reactive oxygen species (ROS): Highly reactive or unstable molecules containing oxygen. A build-up of reactive oxygen species in cells is harmful.

Saturated fats: Saturated fats have no double bonds between carbon molecules because they are saturated with hydrogen molecules, are solid at room temperature and are mainly found in animal products such as butter, lard, meat fat, but also in a few plant foods such as coconut, coconut oil, palm oil, and palm kernel oil.

Semen analysis: The microscopic examination of semen (the male ejaculate) to determine its volume, the number of sperm (sperm count), their shapes (morphology), and their ability to move (motility) in addition to other parameters.

Semen: A mixture of sperm and secretions of sexual accessory glands such as lipids, proteins, glycans and inorganic ions.

Sperm Concentration: Normal sperm concentrations range from 15 million to greater than 200 million sperm per milliliter (mL) of semen. Fewer than 15 million sperm per mL of semen is considered a low sperm count and can interfere with conceiving.

Sperm morphology: The size and shape of sperm.

Sperm motility: The ability of sperm to swim efficiently to fertilize an egg, measured by swimming ability and speed.

Sperm: Male reproductive cells produced by the testes that fertilize a woman's egg.

Spermatogenesis: The biological process of forming mature sperm cells that occurs in the male gonad.

Spina bifida: A birth defect that occurs when the spine and spinal cord don't form properly.

Stillbirth: The death or loss of a baby before or during delivery. Both miscarriage and stillbirth describe pregnancy loss, but they differ according to when the loss occurs.

Synbiotic: A mixture comprising live microorganisms and substrate(s) selectively utilized by host microorganisms that confers a health benefit on the host.

Taxa: The plural of taxon, which is any unit used in the science of biological classification, or taxonomy. Taxa are arranged in a hierarchy from kingdom to subspecies.

Telomere: The natural end of a chromosome composed of a usually repetitive DNA sequence and serving to stabilize the chromosome.

Teratozoospermia: Abnormal sperm shape.

Testes: The two male reproductive glands located in the scrotum, which produce testosterone and sperm.

Testosterone: The primary male hormone produced by the testes that is responsible for the production of sperm, male physical characteristics, and sex drive. Testosterone is also produced in small quantities by the ovaries in women.

Trans fats: Hydrogenated vegetable oils, ubiquitous in margarine and shortenings at one time but now almost phased out of the Western food supply. Trans fats may increase the risk of heart disease, diabetes and inflammation.

Unsaturated fatty acids: Contain one or more double bonds and include omega-3 fatty acids such as DHA, EPA, and α-linolenic acid; omega-6 fatty acids such as linoleic acid and γ-linolenic acid; and omega-9 fatty acids such as oleic acid.

Uterus: The hollow, muscular organ in a woman's pelvis where an embryo implants and grows during pregnancy. Also called the womb.

BIBLIOGRAPHY

"The Menstrual Cycle and Ovulation." *Marin Fertility Center*, 2021, marinfertilitycenter.com/new-getting-started/infertility-basics/.

WHO Expert Consultation. "Appropriate body-mass index for Asian populations and its implications for policy and intervention strategies." Lancet (London, England) vol. 363,9403 (2004): 157-63. doi:10.1016/S0140-6736(03)15268-3

Adams, James B et al. "Evidence-Based Recommendations for an Optimal Prenatal Supplement for Women in the U.S., Part Two: Minerals." *Nutrients* vol. 13,6 1849. 28 May. 2021, doi:10.3390/nu13061849

Afeiche, M et al. "Dairy food intake in relation to semen quality and reproductive hormone levels among physically active young men." *Human reproduction (Oxford, England)* vol. 28, 8 (2013): 2265-75. doi:10.1093/humrep/det133

Afeiche, Myriam C et al. "Dairy intake and semen quality among men attending a fertility clinic." *Fertility and sterility* vol. 101, 5 (2014): 1280-7. doi:10.1016/j.fertnstert.2014.02.003

Agarwal, Ashok et al. "Male Oxidative Stress Infertility (MOSI): Proposed Terminology and Clinical Practice Guidelines for Management of Idiopathic Male Infertility." *The world journal of men's health* vol. 37,3 (2019): 296-312. doi:10.5534/wjmh.190055

Agarwal, Ashok et al. "Role of antioxidants in treatment of male infertility: an overview of the literature." *Reproductive biomedicine online* vol. 8,6 (2004): 616-27. doi:10.1016/s1472-6483(10)61641-0

Agarwal, Ashok et al. "The effects of oxidative stress on female reproduction: a review." *Reproductive biology and endocrinology : RB&E* vol. 10 49. 29 Jun. 2012, doi:10.1186/1477-7827-10-49

Agarwal, Ashok et al. "Utility of Antioxidants in the Treatment of Male Infertility: Clinical Guidelines Based on a Systematic Review and Analysis of Evidence." *The world journal of men's health* vol. 39,2 (2021): 233-290. doi:10.5534/wjmh.200196

Agostoni, Carlo et al. "Whole blood fatty acid composition at birth: from the maternal compartment to the infant." *Clinical nutrition (Edinburgh, Scotland)* vol. 30,4 (2011): 503-5. doi:10.1016/j.clnu.2011.01.016

Agrawal, Rina et al. "Prospective randomized trial of multiple micronutrients in subfertile women undergoing ovulation induction: a pilot study." Reproductive biomedicine online vol. 24,1 (2012): 54-60. doi:10.1016/j.rbmo.2011.10.004

Al-Safi, Zain A et al. "Omega-3 Fatty Acid Supplementation Lowers Serum FSH in Normal Weight But Not Obese Women." The Journal of clinical endocrinology and metabolism vol. 101,1 (2016): 324-33. doi:10.1210/jc.2015-2913

Aldunate, Muriel et al. "Antimicrobial and immune modulatory effects of lactic acid and short chain fatty acids produced by vaginal microbiota associated with eubiosis and bacterial vaginosis." *Frontiers in physiology* vol. 6 164. 2 Jun. 2015, doi:10.3389/fphys.2015.00164

Altmäe, Signe et al. "The seminal microbiome in health and disease." *Nature reviews. Urology* vol. 16,12 (2019): 703-721. doi:10.1038/s41585-019-0250-y

Altmäe, Signe. "Commentary: Uterine Microbiota: Residents, Tourists, or Invaders?" *Frontiers in immunology* vol. 9 1874. 24 Aug. 2018, doi:10.3389/fimmu.2018.01874

Amin, Ahmed F et al. "N-acetyl cysteine for treatment of recurrent unexplained pregnancy loss." *Reproductive biomedicine online* vol. 17,5 (2008): 722-6. doi:10.1016/s1472-6483(10)60322-7

Amiri Siavashani, Mehrnush et al. "The Effects of Chromium Supplementation on Gene Expression of Insulin, Lipid, and Inflammatory Markers in Infertile Women With Polycystic Ovary Syndrome Candidate for *in vitro* Fertilization: A Randomized, Double-Blinded, Placebo-Controlled Trial." *Frontiers in endocrinology* vol. 9 726. 28 Nov. 2018, doi:10.3389/fendo.2018.00726

Anahtar, Melis N et al. "Cervicovaginal Microbiota and Reproductive Health: The Virtue of Simplicity." *Cell host & microbe* vol. 23,2 (2018): 159-168. doi:10.1016/j.chom.2018.01.013

Anahtar, Melis N et al. "Cervicovaginal Microbiota and Reproductive Health: The Virtue of Simplicity." *Cell host &*

microbe vol. 23,2 (2018): 159-168. doi:10.1016/j.chom.2018.01.013

Angulo, Constanza et al. "Vitamin C and oxidative stress in the seminiferous epithelium." Biological research vol. 44,2 (2011): 169-80.

Anukam, Kingsley C et al. "Clinical study comparing probiotic Lactobacillus GR-1 and RC-14 with metronidazole vaginal gel to treat symptomatic bacterial vaginosis." *Microbes and infection* vol. 8,12-13 (2006): 2772-6. doi:10.1016/j.micinf.2006.08.008

Archana, D et al. "Alleviative effect of resveratrol on polyvinyl chloride-induced reproductive toxicity in male Wistar rats." Food and chemical toxicology : an international journal published for the British Industrial Biological Research Association vol. 116,Pt B (2018): 173-181. doi:10.1016/j.fct.2018.04.026

Asa, Elham et al. "Supplementation of freezing media with alpha lipoic acid preserves the structural and functional characteristics of sperm against cryodamage in infertile men with asthenoteratozoospermia." Cryobiology vol. 96 (2020): 166-174. doi:10.1016/j.cryobiol.2020.07.001

Atanasovska, Emilija et al. "Vitamin D levels and oxidative stress markers in patients hospitalized with COVID-19." *Redox report : communications in free radical research* vol. 26,1 (2021): 184-189. doi:10.1080/13510002.2021.1999126

Attaman, Jill A et al. "Dietary fat and semen quality among men attending a fertility clinic." *Human reproduction (Oxford, England)* vol. 27,5 (2012): 1466-74. doi:10.1093/humrep/des065

Awad, Hosni et al. "Melatonin hormone profile in infertile males." International journal of andrology vol. 29,3 (2006): 409-13. doi:10.1111/j.1365-2605.2005.00624.x

Badawy, Ahmed et al. "N-Acetyl cysteine and clomiphene citrate for induction of ovulation in polycystic ovary syndrome: a cross-over trial." *Acta obstetricia et gynecologica Scandinavica* vol. 86,2 (2007): 218-22. doi:10.1080/00016340601090337

Bagnall, Paulette, and Denise Rizzolo. "Bacterial vaginosis: A practical review." *JAAPA : official journal of the American Academy of Physician Assistants* vol. 30,12 (2017): 15-21. doi:10.1097/01.JAA.0000526770.60197.fa

Balercia, G et al. "Coenzyme Q10 and male infertility." Journal of endocrinological investigation vol. 32,7 (2009): 626-32. doi:10.1007/BF03346521

Balogun, Olukunmi O et al. "Vitamin supplementation for preventing miscarriage." The Cochrane database of systematic reviews vol. 2016,5 CD004073. 6 May. 2016, doi:10.1002/14651858.CD004073.pub4

Banaszewska, Beata et al. "Effects of Resveratrol on Polycystic Ovary Syndrome: A Double-blind, Randomized, Placebo-controlled Trial." *The Journal of clinical endocrinology and metabolism* vol. 101,11 (2016): 4322-4328. doi:10.1210/jc.2016-1858

Banihani, Saleem Ali. "Vitamin B_{12} and Semen Quality." *Biomolecules* vol. 7,2 42. 9 Jun. 2017, doi:10.3390/biom7020042

Barbonetti, Arcangelo et al. "Effect of vaginal probiotic lactobacilli on in vitro-induced sperm lipid peroxidation and its impact on sperm motility and viability." *Fertility and sterility* vol. 95,8 (2011): 2485-8. doi:10.1016/j.fertnstert.2011.03.066

Beltrame, Flávia Luciana et al. "Vitamin B_{12} Prevents Cimetidine-Induced Androgenic Failure and Damage to Sperm Quality in Rats." *Frontiers in endocrinology* vol. 10 309. 10 Jul. 2019, doi:10.3389/fendo.2019.00309

Benner, Marilen et al. "How uterine microbiota might be responsible for a receptive, fertile endometrium." *Human reproduction update* vol. 24,4 (2018): 393-415. doi:10.1093/humupd/dmy012

Bennett, M. "Vitamin B12 deficiency, infertility and recurrent fetal loss." *The Journal of reproductive medicine* vol. 46,3 (2001): 209-12.

Bentov, Yaakov et al. "Coenzyme Q10 Supplementation and Oocyte Aneuploidy in Women Undergoing IVF-ICSI Treatment." *Clinical medicine insights. Reproductive health* vol. 8 31-6. 8 Jun. 2014, doi:10.4137/CMRH.S14681

Best, Damian et al. "How effective are weight-loss interventions for improving fertility in women and men who are overweight or obese? A systematic review and meta-analysis of the evidence." *Human reproduction update* vol. 23,6 (2017): 681-705. doi:10.1093/humupd/dmx027

Bhandari, Praveen, and Vijay Prabha. "Evaluation of profertility effect of probiotic Lactobacillus plantarum 2621 in a murine model." *The Indian journal of medical research* vol. 142,1 (2015): 79-84. doi:10.4103/0971-5916.162127

Bieniek, Jared M et al. "Influence of increasing body mass index on semen and reproductive hormonal parameters in a multi-institutional cohort of subfertile men." *Fertility and sterility* vol. 106,5 (2016): 1070-1075. doi:10.1016/j.fertnstert.2016.06.041

Bieniek, Jared M, and Kirk C Lo. "Recent advances in understanding & managing male infertility." *F1000Research* vol. 5 2756. 24 Nov. 2016, doi:10.12688/f1000research.9375.1

Biviá-Roig, Gemma et al. "Impact of the COVID-19 Pandemic on the Lifestyles and Quality of Life of Women With Fertility Problems: A Cross-Sectional Study." Frontiers in public health vol. 9 686115. 19 Jul. 2021, doi:10.3389/fpubh.2021.686115

Bleau, G et al. "Semen selenium and human fertility." Fertility and sterility vol. 42,6 (1984): 890-4.

Bohbot, J M et al. "Efficacy and safety of vaginally administered lyophilized Lactobacillus crispatus IP 174178 in the prevention of bacterial vaginosis recurrence." *Journal of gynecology obstetrics and human reproduction* vol. 47,2 (2018): 81-86. doi:10.1016/j.jogoh.2017.11.005

Boutari, Chrysoula et al. "The effect of underweight on female and male reproduction." Metabolism: clinical and experimental vol. 107 (2020): 154229. doi:10.1016/j.metabol.2020.154229

Boxmeer, Jolanda C et al. "Low folate in seminal plasma is associated with increased sperm DNA damage." *Fertility and sterility* vol. 92,2 (2009): 548-56. doi:10.1016/j.fertnstert.2008.06.010

Bradshaw, Catriona S et al. "High recurrence rates of bacterial vaginosis over the course of 12 months after oral metronidazole therapy and factors associated with recurrence." *The Journal of infectious diseases* vol. 193,11 (2006): 1478-86. doi:10.1086/503780

Braga, Daniela Paes Almeida Ferreira et al. "The impact of food intake and social habits on embryo quality and the likelihood of blastocyst formation." *Reproductive biomedicine online* vol. 31,1 (2015): 30-8. doi:10.1016/j.rbmo.2015.03.007

Brotman, Rebecca M et al. "The effect of vaginal douching cessation on bacterial vaginosis: a pilot study." *American journal of obstetrics and gynecology* vol. 198,6 (2008): 628.e1-7. doi:10.1016/j.ajog.2007.11.043

Broughton, Darcy E, and Kelle H Moley. "Obesity and female infertility: potential mediators of obesity's impact." *Fertility and sterility* vol. 107,4 (2017): 840-847. doi:10.1016/j.fertnstert.2017.01.017

Budani, Maria Cristina, and Gian Mario Tiboni. "Effects of Supplementation with Natural Antioxidants on Oocytes and Preimplantation Embryos." Antioxidants (Basel, Switzerland) vol. 9,7 612. 12 Jul. 2020, doi:10.3390/antiox9070612

Bulik, C M et al. "Fertility and reproduction in women with anorexia nervosa: a controlled study." The Journal of clinical psychiatry vol. 60,2 (1999): 130-5; quiz 135-7. doi:10.4088/jcp.v60n0212

Cai, Hui et al. "Responses and coping methods of different testicular cell types to heat stress: overview and perspectives." *Bioscience reports* vol. 41,6 (2021): BSR20210443. doi:10.1042/BSR20210443

Campisciano, Giuseppina et al. "Subclinical alteration of the cervical-vaginal microbiome in women with idiopathic infertility." *Journal of cellular physiology* vol. 232,7 (2017): 1681-1688. doi:10.1002/jcp.25806

Cannarella, Rossella et al. "Effects of Selenium Supplementation on Sperm Parameters and DNA-Fragmentation Rate in Patients with Chronic Autoimmune Thyroiditis." Journal of clinical medicine vol. 10,16 3755. 23 Aug. 2021, doi:10.3390/jcm10163755

Cánovas-Conesa, A et al. "The association of adherence to a Mediterranean diet during early pregnancy and the risk of gastroschisis in the offspring." *Cirugia pediatrica : organo oficial de la Sociedad Espanola de Cirugia Pediatrica* vol. 26,1 (2013): 37-43.

Cariati, Federica et al. "Bisphenol a: an emerging threat to male fertility". *Reproductive biology and endocrinology : RB&E* vol. 17,1 6. 20 Jan. 2019, doi:10.1186/s12958-018-0447-6

Cariati, Federica et al. "The evolving role of genetic tests in reproductive medicine." Journal of translational medicine vol. 17,1 267. 14 Aug. 2019, doi:10.1186/s12967-019-2019-8

Carlomagno, G, and V Unfer. "Inositol safety: clinical evidences." *European review for medical and pharmacological sciences* vol. 15,8 (2011): 931-6.

Carlsen, E et al. "Evidence for decreasing quality of semen during past 50 years." BMJ (Clinical research ed.) vol. 305,6854 (1992): 609-13. doi:10.1136/bmj.305.6854.609

Caronia, Lisa M et al. "Abrupt decrease in serum testosterone levels after an oral glucose load in men: implications for screening for hypogonadism." Clinical endocrinology vol. 78,2 (2013): 291-6. doi:10.1111/j.1365-2265.2012.04486.x

Carroll, K et al. "Marijuana use and its influence on sperm morphology and motility: identified risk for fertility among Jamaican men." *Andrology* vol. 8,1 (2020): 136-142. doi:10.1111/andr.12670

Casilla-Lennon, Marianne M et al. "The effect of antidepressants on fertility." *American journal of obstetrics and gynecology* vol. 215,3 (2016): 314.e1-5. doi:10.1016/j.ajog.2016.01.170

Cavallini, Giorgio. "Male idiopathic oligoasthenoteratozoospermia." *Asian journal of andrology* vol. 8,2 (2006): 143-57. doi:10.1111/j.1745-7262.2006.00123.x

Cetin, I et al. "Role of micronutrients in the periconceptional period." *Human reproduction update* vol. 16,1 (2010): 80-95. doi:10.1093/humupd/dmp025

Chaer, Rayane et al. "Fertility and Reproduction after Recovery from Anorexia Nervosa: A Systematic Review and Meta-Analysis of Long-Term Follow-Up Studies." Diseases (Basel, Switzerland) vol. 8,4 46. 16 Dec. 2020, doi:10.3390/diseases8040046

Chang, Catherine et al. "The Impact of Bariatric Surgery Compared to Metformin Therapy on Pregnancy Outcomes in Patients with Polycystic Ovarian Syndrome: a Systematic Review and Meta-analysis." Journal of gastrointestinal surgery: official journal of the Society for Surgery of the Alimentary Tract vol. 25,2 (2021): 378-386. doi:10.1007/s11605-020-04900-3

Chavarro, J E et al. "A prospective study of dairy foods intake and anovulatory infertility." *Human reproduction (Oxford, England)* vol. 22,5 (2007): 1340-7. doi:10.1093/humrep/dem019

Chavarro, Jorge E et al. "Body mass index and short-term weight change in relation to treatment outcomes in women undergoing assisted reproduction." *Fertility and sterility* vol. 98,1 (2012): 109-16. doi:10.1016/j.fertnstert.2012.04.012

Chavarro, Jorge E et al. "Diet and lifestyle in the prevention of ovulatory disorder infertility." *Obstetrics and gynecology* vol. 110,5 (2007): 1050-8. doi:10.1097/01.AOG.0000287293.25465.e1

Chavarro, J E et al. "A prospective study of dairy foods intake and anovulatory infertility." *Human reproduction (Oxford, England)* vol. 22,5 (2007): 1340-7. doi:10.1093/humrep/dem019

Chavarro, Jorge E et al. "Soy food and isoflavone intake in relation to semen quality parameters among men from an infertility clinic." *Human reproduction (Oxford, England)* vol. 23,11 (2008): 2584-90. doi:10.1093/humrep/den243

Chavarro, J E et al. "A prospective study of dietary carbohydrate quantity and quality in relation to risk of ovulatory infertility." European journal of clinical nutrition vol. 63,1 (2009): 78-86. doi:10.1038/sj.ejcn.1602904

Chavarro, Jorge E et al. "Protein intake and ovulatory infertility." *American journal of obstetrics and gynecology* vol. 198,2 (2008): 210.e1-7. doi:10.1016/j.ajog.2007.06.057

Chavarro, Jorge E et al. "Dietary fatty acid intakes and the risk of ovulatory infertility." *The American journal of clinical nutrition* vol. 85,1 (2007): 231-7. doi:10.1093/ajcn/85.1.231

Chavarro, J.E. et al. "Dietary fat intake and in-vitro fertilization outcomes: saturated fat intake is associated with fewer metaphase 2 oocytes." *Human Reproduction*, Volume 27, Issue suppl_2, 2012, Pages ii78–ii79, https://doi.org/10.1093/humrep/27.s2.52

Chavarro, Jorge E et al. "Trans-fatty acid levels in sperm are associated with sperm concentration among men from an infertility clinic." *Fertility and sterility* vol. 95,5 (2011): 1794-7. doi:10.1016/j.fertnstert.2010.10.039

Chen, Chen et al. "The microbiota continuum along the female reproductive tract and its relation to uterine-related diseases." *Nature communications* vol. 8,1 875. 17 Oct. 2017, doi:10.1038/s41467-017-00901-0

Chen, X L et al. "Antioxidative activity and protective effect of probiotics against high-fat diet-induced sperm damage in rats." *Animal : an international journal of animal bioscience* vol. 7,2 (2013): 287-92. doi:10.1017/S1751731112001528

Chiu, Y H et al. "Sugar-sweetened beverage intake in relation to semen quality and reproductive hormone levels in young men." *Human reproduction (Oxford, England)* vol. 29,7 (2014): 1575-84. doi:10.1093/humrep/deu102

Chiu, Y-H et al. "Serum omega-3 fatty acids and treatment outcomes among women undergoing assisted reproduction." *Human reproduction (Oxford, England)* vol. 33,1 (2018): 156-165. doi:10.1093/humrep/dex335

Chu, Justin et al. "Vitamin D and assisted reproductive treatment outcome: a systematic review and meta-analysis." *Human reproduction (Oxford, England)* vol. 33,1 (2018): 65-80. doi:10.1093/humrep/dex326

Cicek, Nedim et al. "Vitamin E effect on controlled ovarian stimulation of unexplained infertile women." *Journal of assisted reproduction and genetics* vol. 29,4 (2012): 325-8. doi:10.1007/s10815-012-9714-1

Cicinelli, Ettore et al. "Chronic endometritis in patients with unexplained infertility: Prevalence and effects of antibiotic treatment on spontaneous conception." *American journal of reproductive immunology (New York, N.Y. : 1989)* vol. 79,1 (2018): 10.1111/aji.12782. doi:10.1111/aji.12782

Cirillo, Michela et al. "The effects of COVID-19 lockdown on lifestyle and emotional state in women undergoing assisted reproductive technology: Results of an Italian survey." Journal of gynecology obstetrics and human reproduction vol. 50,8 (2021): 102079. doi:10.1016/j.jogoh.2021.102079

Cito, Gianmartin et al. "Vitamin D and Male Fertility: An Updated Review." *The world journal of men's health* vol. 38,2 (2020): 164-177. doi:10.5534/wjmh.190057

Claustrat, B, and J Leston. "Melatonin: Physiological effects in humans." Neuro-Chirurgie vol. 61,2-3 (2015): 77-84. doi:10.1016/j.neuchi.2015.03.002

Collodel, Giulia et al. "Relevance of Fatty Acids to Sperm Maturation and Quality." *Oxidative medicine and cellular longevity* vol. 2020 7038124. 5 Feb. 2020, doi:10.1155/2020/7038124

Corbett, G A et al. "Probiotic therapy in couples with infertility: A systematic review." *European journal of obstetrics, gynecology, and reproductive biology* vol. 256 (2021): 95-100. doi:10.1016/j.ejogrb.2020.10.054

Cueto, H T et al. "Folic acid supplementation and fecundability: a Danish prospective cohort study." *European journal of clinical nutrition* vol. 70,1 (2016): 66-71. doi:10.1038/ejcn.2015.94

Cutillas-Tolín, A et al. "Mediterranean and western dietary patterns are related to markers of testicular function among healthy men." *Human reproduction (Oxford, England)* vol. 30,12 (2015): 2945-55. doi:10.1093/humrep/dev236

Dardmeh, Fereshteh et al. "Lactobacillus rhamnosus PB01 (DSM 14870) supplementation affects markers of sperm kinematic parameters in a diet-induced obesity mice model." *PloS one* vol. 12,10 e0185964. 10 Oct. 2017, doi:10.1371/journal.pone.0185964

D'Argenio, Valeria. "The Prenatal Microbiome: A New Player for Human Health." *High-throughput* vol. 7,4 38. 11 Dec. 2018, doi:10.3390/ht7040038

de Angelis, Cristina et al. "The role of vitamin D in male fertility: A focus on the testis." Reviews in endocrine & metabolic disorders vol. 18,3 (2017): 285-305. doi:10.1007/s11154-017-9425-0

De Luca, Maria Nunzia et al. "Oxidative Stress and Male Fertility: Role of Antioxidants and Inositols." Antioxidants (Basel, Switzerland) vol. 10,8 1283. 13 Aug. 2021, doi:10.3390/antiox10081283

Desai, Nisarg et al. "Free radical theory of aging: implications in male infertility." *Urology* vol. 75,1 (2010): 14-9. doi:10.1016/j.urology.2009.05.025

Di Tucci, Chiara et al. "The role of alpha lipoic acid in female and male infertility: a systematic review." *Gynecological endocrinology: the official journal of the International Society of*

Gynecological Endocrinology vol. 37,6 (2021): 497-505. doi:10.1080/09513590.2020.1843619

Ding, Jiayi et al. "FDA-approved medications that impair human spermatogenesis." *Oncotarget* vol. 8,6 (2017): 10714-10725. doi:10.18632/oncotarget.12956

Domar, A D et al. "Impact of group psychological interventions on pregnancy rates in infertile women." *Fertility and sterility* vol. 73,4 (2000): 805-11. doi:10.1016/s0015-0282(99)00493-8

Drakopoulos, Panagiotis et al. "The effect of serum vitamin D levels on ovarian reserve markers: a prospective cross-sectional study." *Human reproduction (Oxford, England)* vol. 32,1 (2017): 208-214. doi:10.1093/humrep/dew304

Drobnis, Erma Z, and Ajay K Nangia. "Pain Medications and Male Reproduction." *Advances in experimental medicine and biology* vol. 1034 (2017): 39-57. doi:10.1007/978-3-319-69535-8_6

Dull, Ana-Maria et al. "Therapeutic Approaches of Resveratrol on Endometriosis via Anti-Inflammatory and Anti-Angiogenic Pathways." *Molecules (Basel, Switzerland)* vol. 24,4 667. 13 Feb. 2019, doi:10.3390/molecules24040667

Ebisch, I M W et al. "Does folic acid and zinc sulphate intervention affect endocrine parameters and sperm characteristics in men?." International journal of andrology vol. 29,2 (2006): 339-45. doi:10.1111/j.1365-2605.2005.00598.x

Ebisch, I M W et al. “The importance of folate, zinc and antioxidants in the pathogenesis and prevention of subfertility.” *Human reproduction update* vol. 13,2 (2007): 163-74. doi:10.1093/humupd/dml054

Efrat, Michal et al. “Dietary patterns are positively associated with semen quality.” Fertility and sterility vol. 109,5 (2018): 809-816. doi:10.1016/j.fertnstert.2018.01.010

Egbase, P E et al. “Incidence of microbial growth from the tip of the embryo transfer catheter after embryo transfer in relation to clinical pregnancy rate following in-vitro fertilization and embryo transfer.” Human reproduction (Oxford, England) vol. 11,8 (1996): 1687-9. doi:10.1093/oxfordjournals.humrep.a019470

Eisenberg, Michael L et al. “Increased risk of incident chronic medical conditions in infertile men: analysis of United States claims data.” *Fertility and sterility* vol. 105,3 (2016): 629-636. doi:10.1016/j.fertnstert.2015.11.011

El Refaeey, Abdelaziz et al. “Combined coenzyme Q10 and clomiphene citrate for ovulation induction in clomiphene-citrate-resistant polycystic ovary syndrome.” Reproductive biomedicine online vol. 29,1 (2014): 119-24. doi:10.1016/j.rbmo.2014.03.011

Elango, Rajavel, and Ronald O Ball. “Protein and Amino Acid Requirements during Pregnancy.” *Advances in nutrition (Bethesda, Md.)* vol. 7,4 839S-44S. 15 Jul. 2016, doi:10.3945/an.115.011817

Erland, Lauren A E, and Praveen K Saxena. "Melatonin Natural Health Products and Supplements: Presence of Serotonin and Significant Variability of Melatonin Content." *Journal of clinical sleep medicine : JCSM : official publication of the American Academy of Sleep Medicine* vol. 13,2 275-281. 15 Feb. 2017, doi:10.5664/jcsm.6462

Eskew, Ashley M et al. "Dietary patterns are associated with improved ovarian reserve in overweight and obese women: a cross-sectional study of the Lifestyle and Ovarian Reserve (LORe) cohort." *Reproductive biology and endocrinology : RB&E* vol. 20,1 33. 19 Feb. 2022, doi:10.1186/s12958-022-00907-4

Escobar-Morreale, Héctor F et al. "The polycystic ovary syndrome associated with morbid obesity may resolve after weight loss induced by bariatric surgery." The Journal of clinical endocrinology and metabolism vol. 90,12 (2005): 6364-9. doi:10.1210/jc.2005-1490

Eslamian, Ghazaleh et al. "Intake of food groups and idiopathic asthenozoospermia: a case-control study." *Human reproduction (Oxford, England)* vol. 27,11 (2012): 3328-36. doi:10.1093/humrep/des311

Fallah, Ali et al. "Zinc is an Essential Element for Male Fertility: A Review of Zn Roles in Men's Health, Germination, Sperm Quality, and Fertilization." Journal of reproduction & infertility vol. 19,2 (2018): 69-81.

Farahani, Linda et al. "The semen microbiome and its impact on sperm function and male fertility: A systematic review and meta-analysis." *Andrology* vol. 9,1 (2021): 115-144. doi:10.1111/andr.12886

Farinha, Juliano Boufleur et al. "Response of oxidative stress and inflammatory biomarkers to a 12-week aerobic exercise training in women with metabolic syndrome." Sports medicine - open vol. 1,1 (2015): 19. doi:10.1186/s40798-015-0011-2

Fernández, Leónides et al. "Application of Ligilactobacillus salivarius CECT5713 to Achieve Term Pregnancies in Women with Repetitive Abortion or Infertility of Unknown Origin by Microbiological and Immunological Modulation of the Vaginal Ecosystem." *Nutrients* vol. 13,1 162. 6 Jan. 2021, doi:10.3390/nu13010162

Florou, Panagiota et al. "Does coenzyme Q_{10} supplementation improve fertility outcomes in women undergoing assisted reproductive technology procedures? A systematic review and meta-analysis of randomized-controlled trials." *Journal of assisted reproduction and genetics* vol. 37,10 (2020): 2377-2387. doi:10.1007/s10815-020-01906-3

Fontana, Roberta, and Sara Della Torre. "The Deep Correlation between Energy Metabolism and Reproduction: A View on the Effects of Nutrition for Women Fertility." *Nutrients* vol. 8,2 87. 11 Feb. 2016, doi:10.3390/nu8020087

Formoso, Gloria et al. "Inositol and antioxidant supplementation: Safety and efficacy in pregnancy."

Diabetes/metabolism research and reviews vol. 35,5 (2019): e3154. doi:10.1002/dmrr.3154

Franasiak, Jason M et al. "Vitamin D levels do not affect IVF outcomes following the transfer of euploid blastocysts." *American journal of obstetrics and gynecology* vol. 212,3 (2015): 315.e1-6. doi:10.1016/j.ajog.2014.09.029

Fui, Mark Ng Tang et al. "Lowered testosterone in male obesity: mechanisms, morbidity and management." *Asian journal of andrology* vol. 16,2 (2014): 223-31. doi:10.4103/1008-682X.122365

Fung, June L et al. "Association of vitamin D intake and serum levels with fertility: results from the Lifestyle and Fertility Study." *Fertility and sterility* vol. 108,2 (2017): 302-311. doi:10.1016/j.fertnstert.2017.05.037

Garcez, Marcia E et al. "Effects of resveratrol supplementation on cryopreservation medium of human semen." Fertility and sterility vol. 94,6 (2010): 2118-21. doi:10.1016/j.fertnstert.2010.01.058

Garcia-Grau, Iolanda et al. "Taxonomical and Functional Assessment of the Endometrial Microbiota in A Context of Recurrent Reproductive Failure: A Case Report." *Pathogens (Basel, Switzerland)* vol. 8,4 205. 24 Oct. 2019, doi:10.3390/pathogens8040205

Garolla, Andrea et al. "Dietary Supplements for Male Infertility: A Critical Evaluation of Their Composition." *Nutrients* vol. 12;5 1472. 19 May. 2020, doi:10.3390/nu12051472

Garruti, Gabriella et al. "Weighing the Impact of Diet and Lifestyle on Female Reproductive Function." Current medicinal chemistry vol. 26,19 (2019): 3584-3592. doi:10.2174/0929867324666170518101008

Gaskins, Audrey J et al. "Association between serum folate and vitamin B-12 and outcomes of assisted reproductive technologies." *The American journal of clinical nutrition* vol. 102,4 (2015): 943-50. doi:10.3945/ajcn.115.112185

Gaskins, Audrey J et al. "Dietary folate and reproductive success among women undergoing assisted reproduction." *Obstetrics and gynecology* vol. 124,4 (2014): 801-809. doi:10.1097/AOG.0000000000000477

Gaskins, Audrey J et al. "Dietary patterns and semen quality in young men." *Human reproduction (Oxford, England)* vol. 27,10 (2012): 2899-907. doi:10.1093/humrep/des298

Gaskins, Audrey J et al. "Maternal prepregnancy folate intake and risk of spontaneous abortion and stillbirth." Obstetrics and gynecology vol. 124,1 (2014): 23-31. doi:10.1097/AOG.0000000000000343

Gaskins, Audrey J et al. "Maternal whole grain intake and outcomes of in vitro fertilization." *Fertility and sterility* vol. 105,6 (2016): 1503-1510.e4. doi:10.1016/j.fertnstert.2016.02.015

Gaskins, Audrey J et al. "Substantial Weight Gain in Adulthood Is Associated with Lower Probability of Live Birth Following Assisted Reproduction." The Journal of nutrition vol. 151, 3 (2021): 649-656. doi:10.1093/jn/nxaa371

Gaskins, Audrey J, and Jorge E Chavarro. "Diet and fertility: a review." *American journal of obstetrics and gynecology* vol. 218,4 (2018): 379-389. doi:10.1016/j.ajog.2017.08.010

Gaskins, Audrey J et al. "Seafood Intake, Sexual Activity, and Time to Pregnancy." *The Journal of clinical endocrinology and metabolism* vol. 103,7 (2018): 2680-2688. doi:10.1210/jc.2018-00385

Gaskins, Audrey J et al. "Dietary patterns and outcomes of assisted reproduction." *American journal of obstetrics and gynecology* vol. 220,6 (2019): 567.e1-567.e18. doi:10.1016/j.ajog.2019.02.004

Ghanei, Nila et al. "The probiotic supplementation reduced inflammation in polycystic ovary syndrome: A randomized, double-blind, placebo-controlled trial."Journal of Functional Foods vol 42 (2018): 306-311, doi.org/10.1016/j.jff.2017.12.047.

Gharagozloo, Parviz, and R John Aitken. "The role of sperm oxidative stress in male infertility and the significance of oral antioxidant therapy." *Human reproduction (Oxford, England)* vol. 26,7 (2011): 1628-40. doi:10.1093/humrep/der132

Gibson, Glenn R et al. "Expert consensus document: The International Scientific Association for Probiotics and Prebiotics (ISAPP) consensus statement on the definition and scope of prebiotics." *Nature reviews. Gastroenterology & hepatology* vol. 14,8 (2017): 491-502. doi:10.1038/nrgastro.2017.75

Gluckman, Peter D, and Mark A Hanson. "Living with the past: evolution, development, and patterns of disease." Science (New York, N.Y.) vol. 305,5691 (2004): 1733-6. doi:10.1126/science.1095292

Gong, Zheng et al. "Lactobacilli inactivate Chlamydia trachomatis through lactic acid but not H2O2." *PloS one* vol. 9,9 e107758. 12 Sep. 2014, doi:10.1371/journal.pone.0107758

Governini, Laura et al. "Respiratory Mitochondrial Efficiency and DNA Oxidation in Human Sperm after In Vitro Myo-Inositol Treatment." Journal of clinical medicine vol. 9,6 1638. 28 May. 2020, doi:10.3390/jcm9061638

Grajecki, Donata et al. "The effect of micronutrient supplements on female fertility: a systematic review." *Archives of gynecology and obstetrics* vol. 285,5 (2012): 1463-71. doi:10.1007/s00404-012-2237-2

Greco, Ermanno et al. "Reduction of the incidence of sperm DNA fragmentation by oral antioxidant treatment." *Journal of andrology* vol. 26,3 (2005): 349-53. doi:10.2164/jandrol.04146

Grieger, Jessica A et al. "Maternal Selenium, Copper and Zinc Concentrations in Early Pregnancy, and the Association with Fertility." *Nutrients* vol. 11,7 1609. 16 Jul. 2019, doi:10.3390/nu11071609

Grodstein, F et al. "Body mass index and ovulatory infertility." Epidemiology (Cambridge, Mass.) vol. 5,2 (1994): 247-50. doi:10.1097/00001648-199403000-00016

Guzmán, Carolina et al. "Maternal protein restriction during pregnancy and/or lactation negatively affects follicular ovarian development and steroidogenesis in the prepubertal rat offspring." Archives of medical research vol. 45,4 (2014): 294-300. doi:10.1016/j.arcmed.2014.05.005

Gvozdjáková, Anna et al. "Coenzyme Q_{10}, α-tocopherol, and oxidative stress could be important metabolic biomarkers of male infertility." Disease markers vol. 2015 (2015): 827941. doi:10.1155/2015/827941

H Hassan, Mohammed et al. "Men with idiopathic oligoasthenoteratozoospermia exhibit lower serum and seminal plasma melatonin levels: Comparative effect of night-light exposure with fertile males." Experimental and therapeutic medicine vol. 20,1 (2020): 235-242. doi:10.3892/etm.2020.8678

Haahr, T et al. "Abnormal vaginal microbiota may be associated with poor reproductive outcomes: a prospective study in IVF patients." *Human reproduction (Oxford, England)* vol. 31,4 (2016): 795-803. doi:10.1093/humrep/dew026

Haghighian, Hossein Khadem et al. "Randomized, triple-blind, placebo-controlled clinical trial examining the effects of alpha-lipoic acid supplement on the spermatogram and seminal oxidative stress in infertile men." *Fertility and sterility* vol. 104,2 (2015): 318-24. doi:10.1016/j.fertnstert.2015.05.014

Håkonsen, Linn Berger et al. "Does weight loss improve semen quality and reproductive hormones? Results from a cohort of severely obese men." *Reproductive health* vol. 8 24. 17 Aug. 2011, doi:10.1186/1742-4755-8-24

Hales, Craig M et al. "Prevalence of Obesity and Severe Obesity Among Adults: United States, 2017-2018." *NCHS data brief* ,360 (2020): 1-8.

Halis, Gülden, and Aydin Arici. "Endometriosis and inflammation in infertility." *Annals of the New York Academy of Sciences* vol. 1034 (2004): 300-15. doi:10.1196/annals.1335.032

Han, Zhen et al. "Maternal underweight and the risk of preterm birth and low birth weight: a systematic review and meta-analyses." International journal of epidemiology vol. 40,1 (2011): 65-101. doi:10.1093/ije/dyq195

Hashan, Mohammad Rashidul et al. "Prevalence and associated factors of underweight, overweight and obesity among women of reproductive age group in the Maldives: Evidence from a nationally representative study." *PloS one* vol. 15,10 e0241621. 29 Oct. 2020, doi:10.1371/journal.pone.0241621

Hashimoto, Tomoko, and Koichi Kyono. "Does dysbiotic endometrium affect blastocyst implantation in IVF patients?." Journal of assisted reproduction and genetics vol. 36,12 (2019): 2471-2479. doi:10.1007/s10815-019-01630-7

Hawkes, Wayne Chris et al. "Selenium supplementation does not affect testicular selenium status or semen quality in North American men." *Journal of andrology* vol. 30,5 (2009): 525-33. doi:10.2164/jandrol.108.006940

Hecht, Leah M et al. "Disordered eating and eating disorders among women seeking fertility treatment: A systematic review." Archives of women's mental health, 10.1007/s00737-021-01156-x. 27 Jun. 2021, doi:10.1007/s00737-021-01156-x

Henkel, Ralf et al. "The excessive use of antioxidant therapy: A possible cause of male infertility?." Andrologia vol. 51,1 (2019): e13162. doi:10.1111/and.13162

Hill, Colin et al. "Expert consensus document. The International Scientific Association for Probiotics and Prebiotics consensus statement on the scope and appropriate use of the term probiotic." Nature reviews. Gastroenterology & hepatology vol. 11,8 (2014): 506-14. doi:10.1038/nrgastro.2014.66

Hoffman, Elizabeth R et al. "Reproductive issues in anorexia nervosa." Expert review of obstetrics & gynecology vol. 6,4 (2011): 403-414. doi:10.1586/eog.11.31

Hogarth, Cathryn A, and Michael D Griswold. "The key role of vitamin A in spermatogenesis." The Journal of clinical investigation vol. 120,4 (2010): 956-62. doi:10.1172/JCI41303

Hohos, Natalie M, and Malgorzata E Skaznik-Wikiel. "High-Fat Diet and Female Fertility." Endocrinology vol. 158,8 (2017): 2407-2419. doi:10.1210/en.2017-00371

Holick, Michael F, and Tai C Chen. "Vitamin D deficiency: a worldwide problem with health consequences." *The American journal of clinical nutrition* vol. 87,4 (2008): 1080S-6S. doi:10.1093/ajcn/87.4.1080S

Holmboe, Stine Agergaard et al. "Use of e-cigarettes associated with lower sperm counts in a cross-sectional study of young men from the general population." *Human reproduction (Oxford, England)* vol. 35,7 (2020): 1693-1701. doi:10.1093/humrep/deaa089

Hosseinzadeh, Pardis et al. "Polycystic Ovary Syndrome and the Forgotten Uterus." F&S reviews vol. 2,1 (2021): 11-20. doi:10.1016/j.xfnr.2020.12.001

Hou, Dongsheng et al. "Microbiota of the seminal fluid from healthy and infertile men." *Fertility and sterility* vol. 100,5 (2013): 1261-9. doi:10.1016/j.fertnstert.2013.07.1991

Hsi, Hsing-Cheng et al. "Methylmercury Concentration in Fish and Risk-Benefit Assessment of Fish Intake among Pregnant versus Infertile Women in Taiwan." *PloS one* vol. 11,5 e0155704. 17 May. 2016, doi:10.1371/journal.pone.0155704

Hu, Kai-Lun et al. "Melatonin Application in Assisted Reproductive Technology: A Systematic Review and Meta-Analysis of Randomized Trials." Frontiers in endocrinology vol. 11 160. 27 Mar. 2020, doi:10.3389/fendo.2020.00160

Huang, Chuan et al. "Decline in semen quality among 30,636 young Chinese men from 2001 to 2015." *Fertility and sterility* vol. 107,1 (2017): 83-88.e2. doi:10.1016/j.fertnstert.2016.09.035

Hyman, Richard W et al. "The dynamics of the vaginal microbiome during infertility therapy with in vitro fertilization-embryo transfer." *Journal of assisted reproduction and genetics* vol. 29,2 (2012): 105-15. doi:10.1007/s10815-011-9694-6

Imterat, Majdi et al. "Impact of Body Mass Index on female fertility and ART outcomes." *Panminerva medica* vol. 61,1 (2019): 58-67. doi:10.23736/S0031-0808.18.03490-0

Irani, Morvarid et al. "The Effect of Folate and Folate Plus Zinc Supplementation on Endocrine Parameters and Sperm Characteristics in Sub-Fertile Men: A Systematic Review and Meta-Analysis." *Urology journal* vol. 14,5 4069-4078. 29 Aug. 2017

Jain, Akas et al. "Pulsatile luteinizing hormone amplitude and progesterone metabolite excretion are reduced in obese women." *The Journal of clinical endocrinology and metabolism* vol. 92,7 (2007): 2468-73. doi:10.1210/jc.2006-2274

Jamilian, Mehri et al. "The Effects of Chromium Supplementation on Endocrine Profiles, Biomarkers of Inflammation, and Oxidative Stress in Women with Polycystic Ovary Syndrome: a Randomized, Double-Blind, Placebo-Controlled Trial." *Biological trace element research* vol. 172,1 (2016): 72-78. doi:10.1007/s12011-015-0570-6

Janas-Kozik, Małgorzata et al. "Systematic Review of Literature on Eating Disorders During Pregnancy-Risk and Consequences for Mother and Child." *Frontiers in psychiatry* vol. 12 777529. 13 Dec. 2021, doi:10.3389/fpsyt.2021.777529

Jensen, Tina K et al. "High dietary intake of saturated fat is associated with reduced semen quality among 701 young

Danish men from the general population." *The American journal of clinical nutrition* vol. 97,2 (2013): 411-8. doi:10.3945/ajcn.112.042432

Jensen, Tina Kold et al. "Associations of Fish Oil Supplement Use With Testicular Function in Young Men." *JAMA network open* vol. 3,1 e1919462. 3 Jan. 2020, doi:10.1001/jamanetworkopen.2019.19462

Jodar, Meritxell et al. "The protein and transcript profiles of human semen." *Cell and tissue research* vol. 363,1 (2016): 85-96. doi:10.1007/s00441-015-2237-1

Johansson, Kari et al. "Outcomes of pregnancy after bariatric surgery." *The New England journal of medicine* vol. 372,9 (2015): 814-24. doi:10.1056/NEJMoa1405789

Jungheim, Emily S et al. "Relationship between serum polyunsaturated fatty acids and pregnancy in women undergoing in vitro fertilization." *The Journal of clinical endocrinology and metabolism* vol. 98,8 (2013): E1364-8. doi:10.1210/jc.2012-4115

Jurewicz, Joanna et al. "Dietary Patterns and Their Relationship With Semen Quality." *American journal of men's health* vol. 12,3 (2018): 575-583. doi:10.1177/1557988315627139

Kadir, Mumta et al. "Folate intake and ovarian reserve among women attending a fertility center." *Fertility and sterility* vol. 117,1 (2022): 171-180. doi:10.1016/j.fertnstert.2021.09.037

Karayiannis, Dimitrios et al. "Adherence to the Mediterranean diet and IVF success rate among non-obese women attempting fertility." *Human reproduction (Oxford, England)* vol. 33,3 (2018): 494-502. doi:10.1093/humrep/dey003

Karayiannis, Dimitrios et al. "Association between adherence to the Mediterranean diet and semen quality parameters in male partners of couples attempting fertility." *Human reproduction (Oxford, England)* vol. 32,1 (2017): 215-222. doi:10.1093/humrep/dew288

Katen, Aimee L et al. "Chronic acrylamide exposure in male mice induces DNA damage to spermatozoa; Potential for amelioration by resveratrol." Reproductive toxicology (Elmsford, N.Y.) vol. 63 (2016): 1-12. doi:10.1016/j.reprotox.2016.05.004

Keller, U et al. "Carnitine status of pregnant women: effect of carnitine supplementation and correlation between iron status and plasma carnitine concentration." *European journal of clinical nutrition* vol. 63,9 (2009): 1098-105. doi:10.1038/ejcn.2009.36

Kessopoulou, E et al. "A double-blind randomized placebo cross-over controlled trial using the antioxidant vitamin E to treat reactive oxygen species associated male infertility." Fertility and sterility vol. 64,4 (1995): 825-31. doi:10.1016/s0015-0282(16)57861-3

Kimmel, M C et al. "Obstetric and gynecologic problems associated with eating disorders." The International journal of eating disorders vol. 49,3 (2016): 260-75. doi:10.1002/eat.22483

Klemmensen, Ak et al. "Intake of vitamin C and E in pregnancy and risk of pre-eclampsia: prospective study among 57 346 women." *BJOG : an international journal of obstetrics and gynaecology* vol. 116,7 (2009): 964-74. doi:10.1111/j.1471-0528.2009.02150.x

Kobori, Yoshitomo et al. "Antioxidant cosupplementation therapy with vitamin C, vitamin E, and coenzyme Q10 in patients with oligoasthenozoospermia." Archivio italiano di urologia, andrologia : organo ufficiale [di] Societa italiana di ecografia urologica e nefrologica vol. 86,1 1-4. 28 Mar. 2014, doi:10.4081/aiua.2014.1.1

Koedooder, Rivka et al. "Identification and evaluation of the microbiome in the female and male reproductive tracts." *Human reproduction update* vol. 25,3 (2019): 298-325. doi:10.1093/humupd/dmy048

Koeth, Robert A et al. "l-Carnitine in omnivorous diets induces an atherogenic gut microbial pathway in humans." *The Journal of clinical investigation* vol. 129,1 (2019): 373-387. doi:10.1172/JCI94601

Koga, Fumitoshi et al. "Relationship between nutrition and reproduction." *Reproductive medicine and biology* vol. 19,3 254-264. 15 Jun. 2020, doi:10.1002/rmb2.12332

Komiya, Shinnosuke et al. "Characterizing the gut microbiota in females with infertility and preliminary results of a water-soluble dietary fiber intervention study." *Journal of clinical biochemistry and nutrition* vol. 67,1 (2020): 105-111. doi:10.3164/jcbn.20-53

Kozopas, Nataliia Mykhailivna et al. "Body Mass Index and Sperm Quality: Is there a Relationship?." *Journal of human reproductive sciences* vol. 13,2 (2020): 110-113. doi:10.4103/jhrs.JHRS_15_20

Ku, Chee Wai et al. "Spontaneous miscarriage in first trimester pregnancy is associated with altered urinary metabolite profile." *BBA clinical* vol. 8 48-55. 19 Aug. 2017, doi:10.1016/j.bbacli.2017.07.003

Kuroda, Keiji et al. "The actions of resveratrol in decidualizing endometrium: acceleration or inhibition?†." *Biology of reproduction* vol. 103,6 (2020): 1152-1156. doi:10.1093/biolre/ioaa172

Kyono, Koichi et al. "Analysis of endometrial microbiota by 16S ribosomal RNA gene sequencing among infertile patients: a single-center pilot study." *Reproductive medicine and biology* vol. 17,3 297-306. 6 May. 2018, doi:10.1002/rmb2.12105

La Vecchia, Irene et al. "Folate, homocysteine and selected vitamins and minerals status in infertile women." *The European journal of contraception & reproductive health care : the official journal of the European Society of Contraception* vol. 22,1 (2017): 70-75. doi:10.1080/13625187.2016.1263292

Lafuente, Rafael et al. "Coenzyme Q10 and male infertility: a meta-analysis." Journal of assisted reproduction and genetics vol. 30,9 (2013): 1147-56. doi:10.1007/s10815-013-0047-5

Lagenaur, Laurel A et al. "Connecting the Dots: Translating the Vaginal Microbiome Into a Drug." *The Journal of infectious diseases* vol. 223,Supplement_3 (2021): S296-S306. doi:10.1093/infdis/jiaa676

Lannon, Sophia M R et al. "Parallel detection of lactobacillus and bacterial vaginosis-associated bacterial DNA in the chorioamnion and vagina of pregnant women at term." *The journal of maternal-fetal & neonatal medicine : the official journal of the European Association of Perinatal Medicine, the Federation of Asia and Oceania Perinatal Societies, the International Society of Perinatal Obstetricians* vol. 32,16 (2019): 2702-2710. doi:10.1080/14767058.2018.1446208

Leary, Christine et al. "Human embryos from overweight and obese women display phenotypic and metabolic abnormalities." *Human reproduction (Oxford, England)* vol. 30,1 (2015): 122-32. doi:10.1093/humrep/deu276

Lefevre, Michael et al. "Comparison of the acute response to meals enriched with cis- or trans-fatty acids on glucose and lipids in overweight individuals with differing FABP2 genotypes." *Metabolism: clinical and experimental* vol. 54,12 (2005): 1652-8. doi:10.1016/j.metabol.2005.06.015

Lerchbaum, Elisabeth, and Barbara Obermayer-Pietsch. "Vitamin D and fertility: a systematic review." *European journal of endocrinology* vol. 166,5 (2012): 765-78. doi:10.1530/EJE-11-0984

Levine, Hagai et al. "Temporal trends in sperm count: a systematic review and meta-regression analysis." *Human reproduction update* vol. 23,6 (2017): 646-659. doi:10.1093/humupd/dmx022

Li, Ming-Chieh et al. "Men's Intake of Vitamin C and β-Carotene Is Positively Related to Fertilization Rate but Not to Live Birth Rate in Couples Undergoing Infertility Treatment." The Journal of nutrition vol. 149,11 (2019): 1977-1984. doi:10.1093/jn/nxz149

Ling, Zongxin et al. "The restoration of the vaginal microbiota after treatment for bacterial vaginosis with metronidazole or probiotics." Microbial ecology vol. 65,3 (2013): 773-80. doi:10.1007/s00248-012-0154-3

Liu, Mengyuan et al. "Resveratrol protects against age-associated infertility in mice." *Human reproduction (Oxford, England)* vol. 28,3 (2013): 707-17. doi:10.1093/humrep/des437

López-Moreno, Ana, and Margarita Aguilera. "Probiotics Dietary Supplementation for Modulating Endocrine and Fertility Microbiota Dysbiosis." *Nutrients* vol. 12,3 757. 13 Mar. 2020, doi:10.3390/nu12030757

López-Moreno, Ana, and Margarita Aguilera. "Vaginal Probiotics for Reproductive Health and Related Dysbiosis: Systematic Review and Meta-Analysis." *Journal of clinical medicine* vol. 10,7 1461. 2 Apr. 2021, doi:10.3390/jcm10071461

Lorenzo, Yolanda et al. "The carotenoid beta-cryptoxanthin stimulates the repair of DNA oxidation damage in addition to acting as an antioxidant in human cells." *Carcinogenesis* vol. 30,2 (2009): 308-14. doi:10.1093/carcin/bgn270

Luddi, Alice et al. "Antioxidants reduce oxidative stress in follicular fluid of aged women undergoing IVF." *Reproductive biology and endocrinology : RB&E* vol. 14,1 57. 7 Sep. 2016, doi:10.1186/s12958-016-0184-7

MacDonald, A A et al. "The impact of body mass index on semen parameters and reproductive hormones in human males: a systematic review with meta-analysis." *Human reproduction update* vol. 16,3 (2010): 293-311. doi:10.1093/humupd/dmp047

Machtinger, Ronit et al. "Association between preconception maternal beverage intake and in vitro fertilization outcomes." Fertility and sterility vol. 108,6 (2017): 1026-1033. doi:10.1016/j.fertnstert.2017.09.007

Madej, Dawid et al. "Influence of Fruit and Vegetable Consumption on Antioxidant Status and Semen Quality: A Cross-Sectional Study in Adult Men." *Frontiers in nutrition* vol. 8 753843. 15 Oct. 2021, doi:10.3389/fnut.2021.753843

Majzoub, Ahmad, and Ashok Agarwal. "Systematic review of antioxidant types and doses in male infertility: Benefits on semen parameters, advanced sperm function, assisted reproduction and live-birth rate." *Arab journal of urology* vol. 16,1 113-124. 2 Jan. 2018, doi:10.1016/j.aju.2017.11.013

Maldonado-Cárceles, Ana B et al. "Dietary patterns and ovarian reserve among women attending a fertility clinic." *Fertility and sterility* vol. 114,3 (2020): 610-617. doi:10.1016/j.fertnstert.2020.04.030

Malmir, Mahdi et al. "Ameliorative effect of melatonin on apoptosis, DNA fragmentation, membrane integrity and lipid peroxidation of spermatozoa in the idiopathic asthenoteratospermic men: In vitro." Andrologia vol. 53,2 (2021): e13944. doi:10.1111/and.13944

Mändar, Reet et al. "Seminal microbiome in men with and without prostatitis." *International journal of urology: official journal of the Japanese Urological Association* vol. 24,3 (2017): 211-216. doi:10.1111/iju.13286

Mändar, Reet et al. "Complementary seminovaginal microbiome in couples." *Research in microbiology* vol. 166,5 (2015): 440-447. doi:10.1016/j.resmic.2015.03.009

Maretti, C, and G Cavallini. "The association of a probiotic with a prebiotic (Flortec, Bracco) to improve the quality/quantity of spermatozoa in infertile patients with idiopathic oligoasthenoteratospermia: a pilot study." *Andrology* vol. 5,3 (2017): 439-444. doi:10.1111/andr.12336

Marić, Tihana et al. "Environmental and occupational exposures associated with male infertility." *Arhiv za higijenu rada i toksikologiju* vol. 72,3 101-113. 28 Jun. 2021, doi:10.2478/aiht-2021-72-3510

Mason, Helen D et al. "Pelvic ultrasonography in anorexia nervosa: what the clinician should ask the radiologist and how to use the information provided." European eating disorders review : the journal of the Eating Disorders Association vol. 15,1 (2007): 35-41. doi:10.1002/erv.719

Mastromarino, P et al. "Effectiveness of Lactobacillus-containing vaginal tablets in the treatment of symptomatic bacterial vaginosis." Clinical microbiology and infection : the official publication of the European Society of Clinical Microbiology and Infectious Diseases vol. 15,1 (2009): 67-74. doi:10.1111/j.1469-0691.2008.02112.x

Mathieu d'Argent, Emmanuelle et al. "High-Dose Supplementation of Folic Acid in Infertile Men Improves IVF-ICSI Outcomes: A Randomized Controlled Trial (FOLFIV Trial)." Journal of clinical medicine vol. 10,9 1876. 26 Apr. 2021, doi:10.3390/jcm10091876

Matthews, T J, and Brady E Hamilton. "Delayed childbearing: more women are having their first child later in life." *NCHS data brief* ,21 (2009): 1-8.

Maya-Enero, Silvia et al. "Neurocognitive and behavioral profile of fetal alcohol spectrum disorder." Anales de pediatria vol. 95,3 (2021): 208.e1-208.e9. doi:10.1016/j.anpede.2020.12.012

Mendiola, Jaime et al. "Food intake and its relationship with semen quality: a case-control study." *Fertility and sterility* vol. 91,3 (2009): 812-8. doi:10.1016/j.fertnstert.2008.01.020

Meng, Xiao et al. "Dietary Sources and Bioactivities of Melatonin." Nutrients vol. 9,4 367. 7 Apr. 2017, doi:10.3390/nu9040367

Merhi, Zaher O et al. "Male adiposity impairs clinical pregnancy rate by in vitro fertilization without affecting day 3 embryo quality." *Obesity (Silver Spring, Md.)* vol. 21,8 (2013): 1608-12. doi:10.1002/oby.20164

Merhi, Zaher O et al. "Circulating vitamin D correlates with serum antimüllerian hormone levels in late-reproductive-aged women: Women's Interagency HIV Study." *Fertility and sterility* vol. 98,1 (2012): 228-34. doi:10.1016/j.fertnstert.2012.03.029

Merviel, Philippe et al. "Impact of myo-inositol treatment in women with polycystic ovary syndrome in assisted reproductive technologies." *Reproductive health* vol. 18,1 13. 19 Jan. 2021, doi:10.1186/s12978-021-01073-3

Mestre Citrinovitz, Ana Cecilia et al. "Resveratrol enhances decidualization of human endometrial stromal cells." *Reproduction (Cambridge, England)* vol. 159,4 (2020): 453-463. doi:10.1530/REP-19-0425

Mikhael, Sasha et al. "Hypothalamic-Pituitary-Ovarian Axis Disorders Impacting Female Fertility." Biomedicines vol. 7,1 5. 4 Jan. 2019, doi:10.3390/biomedicines7010005

Mínguez-Alarcón, Lidia et al. "Dietary intake of antioxidant nutrients is associated with semen quality in young university students." *Human reproduction (Oxford, England)* vol. 27,9 (2012): 2807-14. doi:10.1093/humrep/des247

Mínguez-Alarcón, Lidia et al. "Fatty acid intake in relation to reproductive hormones and testicular volume among young healthy men." *Asian journal of andrology* vol. 19,2 (2017): 184-190. doi:10.4103/1008-682X.190323

Mir, J et al. "Impact of weight loss on sperm DNA integrity in obese men." *Andrologia*, 10.1111/and.12957. 1 Feb. 2018, doi:10.1111/and.12957

Monari, Francesca et al. "Effect of L-Arginine supplementation in pregnant women with chronic hypertension and previous placenta vascular disorders receiving Aspirin prophylaxis: a randomized control trial." *Minerva obstetrics and gynecology*, 10.23736/S2724-606X.21.04827-2. 12 May. 2021, doi:10.23736/S2724-606X.21.04827-2

Monteiro, Catarina et al. "Characterization of microbiota in male infertility cases uncovers differences in seminal hyperviscosity and oligoasthenoteratozoospermia possibly correlated with increased prevalence of infectious bacteria." *American journal of reproductive immunology (New York, N.Y. : 1989)* vol. 79,6 (2018): e12838. doi:10.1111/aji.12838

Moreira-Pinto, Beatriz et al. "Low Doses of Resveratrol Protect Human Granulosa Cells from Induced-Oxidative Stress." *Antioxidants (Basel, Switzerland)* vol. 10,4 561. 4 Apr. 2021, doi:10.3390/antiox10040561

Moreno, Inmaculada et al. "Endometrial microbiota composition is associated with reproductive outcome in infertile patients." *Microbiome* vol. 10,1 1. 4 Jan. 2022, doi:10.1186/s40168-021-01184-w

Moreno, Inmaculada et al. "Evidence that the endometrial microbiota has an effect on implantation success or failure." *American journal of obstetrics and gynecology* vol. 215,6 (2016): 684-703. doi:10.1016/j.ajog.2016.09.075

Moreno, Inmaculada, and Carlos Simon. "Deciphering the effect of reproductive tract microbiota on human reproduction." *Reproductive medicine and biology* vol. 18,1 40-50. 1 Nov. 2018, doi:10.1002/rmb2.12249

Moreno, Inmaculada, and Jason M Franasiak. "Endometrial microbiota-new player in town." *Fertility and sterility* vol. 108,1 (2017): 32-39. doi:10.1016/j.fertnstert.2017.05.034

Moretti, Elena et al. "The presence of bacteria species in semen and sperm quality." *Journal of assisted reproduction and genetics* vol. 26,1 (2009): 47-56. doi:10.1007/s10815-008-9283-5

Mori, Rintaro et al. "Zinc supplementation for improving pregnancy and infant outcome." *The Cochrane database of systematic reviews* ,7 CD000230. 11 Jul. 2012, doi:10.1002/14651858.CD000230.pub4

Moslemi, Mohammad K, and Samaneh Tavanbakhsh. "Selenium-vitamin E supplementation in infertile men: effects on semen parameters and pregnancy rate." *International journal of general medicine* vol. 4 99-104. 23 Jan. 2011, doi:10.2147/IJGM.S16275

Mousa, Aya et al. "Macronutrient and Micronutrient Intake during Pregnancy: An Overview of Recent Evidence." *Nutrients* vol. 11,2 443. 20 Feb. 2019, doi:10.3390/nu11020443

Mozaffarian, Dariush. "Dietary and Policy Priorities for Cardiovascular Disease, Diabetes, and Obesity: A Comprehensive Review." Circulation vol. 133,2 (2016): 187-225. doi:10.1161/CIRCULATIONAHA.115.018585

Mueller, B A et al. "Recreational drug use and the risk of primary infertility." Epidemiology (Cambridge, Mass.) vol. 1,3 (1990): 195-200. doi:10.1097/00001648-199005000-00003

Mumford, S. L., A. Alohali, and J. Wactawski-Wende. "Dietary protein intake and reproductive hormones and ovulation: the BioCycle study." *Fertility and Sterility* 104.3 (2015): e2.

Mumford, Sunni L et al. "Preconception Plasma Phospholipid Fatty Acids and Fecundability." *The Journal of clinical endocrinology and metabolism* vol. 103,12 (2018): 4501-4510. doi:10.1210/jc.2018-00448

Mutsaerts, Meike A Q et al. "Randomized Trial of a Lifestyle Program in Obese Infertile Women." *The New England journal of medicine* vol. 374,20 (2016): 1942-53. doi:10.1056/NEJMoa1505297

Nassan, Feiby L et al. "Diet and men's fertility: does diet affect sperm quality?" *Fertility and sterility* vol. 110,4 (2018): 570-577. doi:10.1016/j.fertnstert.2018.05.025

Nguyen, Ruby H N et al. "Men's body mass index and infertility." *Human reproduction (Oxford, England)* vol. 22,9 (2007): 2488-93. doi:10.1093/humrep/dem139

Nordkap, Loa et al. "Psychological stress and testicular function: a cross-sectional study of 1,215 Danish men." *Fertility and sterility* vol. 105,1 (2016): 174-87.e1-2. doi:10.1016/j.fertnstert.2015.09.016

Nouri, Kazem et al. "The Impact of a Standardized Oral Multinutrient Supplementation on Embryo Quality in in vitro Fertilization/Intracytoplasmic Sperm Injection: A Prospective Randomized Trial." *Gynecologic and obstetric investigation* vol. 82,1 (2017): 8-14. doi:10.1159/000452662

Nouri, Mehran et al. "The effects of lycopene supplement on the spermatogram and seminal oxidative stress in infertile men: A randomized, double-blind, placebo-controlled clinical trial." Phytotherapy research : PTR vol. 33,12 (2019): 3203-3211. doi:10.1002/ptr.6493

Ochiai, Asako et al. "Influence of resveratrol supplementation on IVF-embryo transfer cycle outcomes." *Reproductive biomedicine online* vol. 39,2 (2019): 205-210. doi:10.1016/j.rbmo.2019.03.205

Ochiai, Asako, and Keiji Kuroda. "Preconception resveratrol intake against infertility: Friend or foe?" *Reproductive medicine and biology* vol. 19,2 107-113. 12 Oct. 2019, doi:10.1002/rmb2.12303

Ohri, Manju, and Vijay Prabha. "Isolation of a sperm-agglutinating factor from Staphylococcus aureus isolated from a woman with unexplained infertility." Fertility and sterility vol. 84,5 (2005): 1539-41. doi:10.1016/j.fertnstert.2005.05.030

Okada, Hidetaka et al. "Decidualization of the human endometrium." Reproductive medicine and biology vol. 17,3 220-227. 1 Feb. 2018, doi:10.1002/rmb2.12088

Omu, A E et al. "Treatment of asthenozoospermia with zinc sulphate: andrological, immunological and obstetric outcome." European journal of obstetrics, gynecology, and reproductive biology vol. 79,2 (1998): 179-84. doi:10.1016/s0301-2115(97)00262-5

Ortega, Israel, and Antoni J Duleba. "Ovarian actions of resveratrol." *Annals of the New York Academy of Sciences* vol. 1348,1 (2015): 86-96. doi:10.1111/nyas.12875

Ota, Kuniaki et al. "Vitamin D deficiency may be a risk factor for recurrent pregnancy losses by increasing cellular immunity and autoimmunity." *Human reproduction (Oxford, England)* vol. 29,2 (2014): 208-19. doi:10.1093/humrep/det424

Ourique, Giovana M et al. "Resveratrol prevents oxidative damage and loss of sperm motility induced by long-term treatment with valproic acid in Wistar rats." Experimental and toxicologic pathology : official journal of the Gesellschaft fur

Toxikologische Pathologie vol. 68,8 (2016): 435-43. doi:10.1016/j.etp.2016.07.001

Palafox-Carlos, Hugo et al. "The role of dietary fiber in the bioaccessibility and bioavailability of fruit and vegetable antioxidants." *Journal of food science* vol. 76,1 (2011): R6-R15. doi:10.1111/j.1750-3841.2010.01957.x

Palmer, Nicole O et al. "Diet and exercise in an obese mouse fed a high-fat diet improve metabolic health and reverse perturbed sperm function." *American journal of physiology. Endocrinology and metabolism* vol. 302,7 (2012): E768-80. doi:10.1152/ajpendo.00401.2011

Palmer, Nicole O et al. "Impact of obesity on male fertility, sperm function and molecular composition." *Spermatogenesis* vol. 2,4 (2012): 253-263. doi:10.4161/spmg.21362

Palomba, Stefano et al. "Physical activity before IVF and ICSI cycles in infertile obese women: an observational cohort study." *Reproductive biomedicine online* vol. 29,1 (2014): 72-9. doi:10.1016/j.rbmo.2014.03.006

Parente, E et al. "Safety of oral alpha-lipoic acid treatment in pregnant women: a retrospective observational study." *European review for medical and pharmacological sciences* vol. 21,18 (2017): 4219-4227.

Pascual, Liliana et al. "Vaginal colonization and activity of the probiotic bacterium Lactobacillus fermentum L23 in a murine model of vaginal tract infection." *Journal of medical microbiology* vol. 59,Pt 3 (2010): 360-364. doi:10.1099/jmm.0.012583-0

Pearce, Karma L, and Kelton Tremellen. "The Effect of Macronutrients on Reproductive Hormones in Overweight and Obese Men: A Pilot Study." *Nutrients* vol. 11,12 3059. 14 Dec. 2019, doi:10.3390/nu11123059

Peebles, Kathryn et al. "High Global Burden and Costs of Bacterial Vaginosis: A Systematic Review and Meta-Analysis." *Sexually transmitted diseases* vol. 46,5 (2019): 304-311. doi:10.1097/OLQ.0000000000000972

Pérez-Torres, Israel et al. "Oxidative Stress, Plant Natural Antioxidants, and Obesity." International journal of molecular sciences vol. 22,4 1786. 11 Feb. 2021, doi:10.3390/ijms22041786

Petrova, Mariya I et al. "Lacticaseibacillus rhamnosus GR-1, a.k.a. Lactobacillus rhamnosus GR-1: Past and Future Perspectives." *Trends in microbiology* vol. 29,8 (2021): 747-761. doi:10.1016/j.tim.2021.03.010

Petrova, Mariya I et al. "Lactobacillus iners: Friend or Foe?." *Trends in microbiology* vol. 25,3 (2017): 182-191. doi:10.1016/j.tim.2016.11.007

Plummer, Erica L et al. "Combined oral and topical antimicrobial therapy for male partners of women with bacterial vaginosis: Acceptability, tolerability and impact on the genital microbiota of couples - A pilot study." *PloS one* vol. 13,1 e0190199. 2 Jan. 2018, doi:10.1371/journal.pone.0190199

Poutahidis, Theofilos et al. “Probiotic microbes sustain youthful serum testosterone levels and testicular size in aging mice.” *PloS one* vol. 9,1 e84877. 2 Jan. 2014, doi:10.1371/journal.pone.0084877

Powell, Anna et al. “Clinicians' Use of Intravaginal Boric Acid Maintenance Therapy for Recurrent Vulvovaginal Candidiasis and Bacterial Vaginosis.” *Sexually transmitted diseases* vol. 46,12 (2019): 810-812. doi:10.1097/OLQ.0000000000001063

Qazi, Izhar Hyder et al. “Selenium, Selenoproteins, and Female Reproduction: A Review.” *Molecules (Basel, Switzerland)* vol. 23,12 3053. 22 Nov. 2018, doi:10.3390/molecules23123053

Qian, Jie et al. “An update on the prevalence of eating disorders in the general population: a systematic review and meta-analysis.” Eating and weight disorders : EWD, 10.1007/s40519-021-01162-z. 8 Apr. 2021, doi:10.1007/s40519-021-01162-z

Qu, Fan et al. “The association between psychological stress and miscarriage: A systematic review and meta-analysis.” *Scientific reports* vol. 7,1 1731. 11 May. 2017, doi:10.1038/s41598-017-01792-3

Radwan, M et al. “Sperm DNA damage-the effect of stress and everyday life factors.” *International journal of impotence research* vol. 28,4 (2016): 148-54. doi:10.1038/ijir.2016.15

Rafiee, Bahare et al. “Comparing the Effectiveness of Dietary Vitamin C and Exercise Interventions on Fertility Parameters in Normal Obese Men.” Urology journal vol. 13,2 2635-9. 16 Apr. 2016

Rago, R et al. "Controlled, prospective, observational study on the efficiency and tolerability of a combination of potential Nrf2-inducing antioxidants and micronutrients as pre-treatment for ICSI in dyspermic patients with previous failure." European review for medical and pharmacological sciences vol. 21,7 (2017): 1645-1652.

Rahimlou, Mehran et al. "Dietary Antioxidant Intake in Relation to Semen Quality Parameters in Infertile Men: a Cross-Sectional Study." *Clinical nutrition research* vol. 8,3 229-237. 25 Jul. 2019, doi:10.7762/cnr.2019.8.3.229

Ramakrishnan, Usha et al. "Effect of women's nutrition before and during early pregnancy on maternal and infant outcomes: a systematic review." *Paediatric and perinatal epidemiology* vol. 26 Suppl 1 (2012): 285-301. doi:10.1111/j.1365-3016.2012.01281.x

Ravel, Jacques et al. "Vaginal microbiome of reproductive-age women." *Proceedings of the National Academy of Sciences of the United States of America* vol. 108 Suppl 1, Suppl 1 (2011): 4680-7. doi:10.1073/pnas.1002611107

Ravel, Jacques et al. "Bacterial vaginosis and its association with infertility, endometritis, and pelvic inflammatory disease." *American journal of obstetrics and gynecology* vol. 224,3 (2021): 251-257. doi:10.1016/j.ajog.2020.10.019

Rayman, Margaret P et al. "Effect of long-term selenium supplementation on mortality: Results from a multiple-dose, randomised controlled trial." *Free radical biology & medicine* vol. 127 (2018): 46-54. doi:10.1016/j.freeradbiomed.2018.02.015

Ricci, E et al. "Dietary habits and semen parameters: a systematic narrative review." *Andrology* vol. 6,1 (2018): 104-116. doi:10.1111/andr.12452

Recine, Nadia et al. "Restoring vaginal microbiota: biological control of bacterial vaginosis. A prospective case-control study using Lactobacillus rhamnosus BMX 54 as adjuvant treatment against bacterial vaginosis." *Archives of gynecology and obstetrics* vol. 293,1 (2016): 101-107. doi:10.1007/s00404-015-3810-2

Rizzo, Anthony E et al. "The Female Reproductive Tract Microbiome-Implications for Gynecologic Cancers and Personalized Medicine." *Journal of personalized medicine* vol. 11,6 546. 11 Jun. 2021, doi:10.3390/jpm11060546

Robker, Rebecca L et al. "Obese women exhibit differences in ovarian metabolites, hormones, and gene expression compared with moderate-weight women." *The Journal of clinical endocrinology and metabolism* vol. 94,5 (2009): 1533-40. doi:10.1210/jc.2008-2648

Rodríguez-Varela, Cristina, and Elena Labarta. "Clinical Application of Antioxidants to Improve Human Oocyte Mitochondrial Function: A Review." *Antioxidants (Basel, Switzerland)* vol. 9,12 1197. 28 Nov. 2020, doi:10.3390/antiox9121197

Ruder, Elizabeth H et al. "Female dietary antioxidant intake and time to pregnancy among couples treated for unexplained infertility." *Fertility and sterility* vol. 101,3 (2014): 759-66. doi:10.1016/j.fertnstert.2013.11.008

Ruder, Elizabeth H et al. "Impact of oxidative stress on female fertility." *Current opinion in obstetrics & gynecology* vol. 21,3 (2009): 219-22. doi:10.1097/gco.0b013e32832924ba

Ruder, Elizabeth H et al. "Oxidative stress and antioxidants: exposure and impact on female fertility." *Human reproduction update* vol. 14,4 (2008): 345-57. doi:10.1093/humupd/dmn011

Rudick, Briana J et al. "Influence of vitamin D levels on in vitro fertilization outcomes in donor-recipient cycles." *Fertility and sterility* vol. 101,2 (2014): 447-52. doi:10.1016/j.fertnstert.2013.10.008

Russo, Michele et al. "Melatonin and Myo-Inositol: Supporting Reproduction from the Oocyte to Birth." *International journal of molecular sciences* vol. 22,16 8433. 5 Aug. 2021, doi:10.3390/ijms22168433

Sadaghiani, Safa et al. "Effect of antioxidant supplements on sperm parameters in infertile male smokers: a single-blinded clinical trial." AIMS public health vol. 7,1 92-99. 11 Feb. 2020, doi:10.3934/publichealth.2020009

Safarinejad, Mohammad Reza, and Shiva Safarinejad. "Efficacy of selenium and/or N-acetyl-cysteine for improving semen parameters in infertile men: a double-blind, placebo controlled, randomized study." *The Journal of urology* vol. 181,2 (2009): 741-51. doi:10.1016/j.juro.2008.10.015

Salas-Huetos, Albert et al. "Dietary patterns, foods and nutrients in male fertility parameters and fecundability: a systematic review of observational studies." Human reproduction update vol. 23,4 (2017): 371-389. doi:10.1093/humupd/dmx006

Salas-Huetos, Albert et al. "Male adiposity, sperm parameters and reproductive hormones: An updated systematic review and collaborative meta-analysis." Obesity reviews : an official journal of the International Association for the Study of Obesity vol. 22,1 (2021): e13082. doi:10.1111/obr.13082

Salehi, Bahare et al. "Resveratrol: A Double-Edged Sword in Health Benefits." Biomedicines vol. 6,3 91. 9 Sep. 2018, doi:10.3390/biomedicines6030091

Santander Ballestín, Sonia et al. "Is Supplementation with Micronutrients Still Necessary during Pregnancy? A Review." *Nutrients* vol. 13,9 3134. 8 Sep. 2021, doi:10.3390/nu13093134

Sarais, Veronica et al. "A Comprehensive Analysis of Body Mass Index Effect on in Vitro Fertilization Outcomes." Nutrients vol. 8,3 109. 23 Feb. 2016, doi:10.3390/nu8030109

Scaruffi, Paola et al. "Oral Antioxidant Treatment of Men Significantly Improves the Reproductive Outcome of IVF Cycles." *Journal of clinical medicine* vol. 10,15 3254. 23 Jul. 2021, doi:10.3390/jcm10153254

Schaefer, Ella, and Deborah Nock. "The Impact of Preconceptional Multiple-Micronutrient Supplementation on Female Fertility." *Clinical medicine insights. Women's health* vol. 12 1179562X19843868. 23 Apr. 2019, doi:10.1177/1179562X19843868

Schisterman, Enrique F et al. "Effect of Folic Acid and Zinc Supplementation in Men on Semen Quality and Live Birth Among Couples Undergoing Infertility Treatment: A Randomized Clinical Trial." *JAMA* vol. 323,1 (2020): 35-48. doi:10.1001/jama.2019.18714

Schlotz, Wolff, and David I W Phillips. "Fetal origins of mental health: evidence and mechanisms." Brain, behavior, and immunity vol. 23,7 (2009): 905-16. doi:10.1016/j.bbi.2009.02.001

Schuchardt, Larissa, and Jan Rupp. "Chlamydia trachomatis as the Cause of Infectious Infertility: Acute, Repetitive or Persistent Long-Term Infection?" *Current topics in microbiology and immunology* vol. 412 (2018): 159-182. doi:10.1007/82_2016_15

Scott, R et al. "The effect of oral selenium supplementation on human sperm motility." *British journal of urology* vol. 82,1 (1998): 76-80. doi:10.1046/j.1464-410x.1998.00683.x

Seckl, Jonathan R, and Megan C Holmes. "Mechanisms of disease: glucocorticoids, their placental metabolism and fetal 'programming' of adult pathophysiology." *Nature clinical practice. Endocrinology & metabolism* vol. 3,6 (2007): 479-88. doi:10.1038/ncpendmet0515

Sermondade, N et al. "BMI in relation to sperm count: an updated systematic review and collaborative meta-analysis." *Human reproduction update* vol. 19,3 (2013): 221-31. doi:10.1093/humupd/dms050

Setti, Amanda Souza et al. "Is there an association between artificial sweetener consumption and assisted reproduction outcomes?." Reproductive biomedicine online vol. 36,2 (2018): 145-153. doi:10.1016/j.rbmo.2017.11.004

Shao, Andrew, and John N Hathcock. "Risk assessment for the amino acids taurine, L-glutamine and L-arginine." *Regulatory toxicology and pharmacology : RTP* vol. 50,3 (2008): 376-99. doi:10.1016/j.yrtph.2008.01.004

Sharma, Rakesh et al. "Lifestyle factors and reproductive health: taking control of your fertility." *Reproductive biology and endocrinology : RB&E* vol. 11 66. 16 Jul. 2013, doi:10.1186/1477-7827-11-66

Showell, Marian G et al. "Antioxidants for female subfertility." *The Cochrane database of systematic reviews* vol. 7,7 CD007807. 28 Jul. 2017, doi:10.1002/14651858.CD007807.pub3

Showell, Marian G et al. "Antioxidants for female subfertility." *The Cochrane database of systematic reviews* vol. 8,8 CD007807. 27 Aug. 2020, doi:10.1002/14651858.CD007807.pub4 (Update)

Sińska, Beata et al. "Znaczenie diety w optymalizacji płodności kobiety" [The diet in improving fertility in women]. *Polski merkuriusz lekarski : organ Polskiego Towarzystwa Lekarskiego* vol. 36,216 (2014): 400-2.

Silvestris, Erica et al. "Nutrition and Female Fertility: An Interdependent Correlation." *Frontiers in endocrinology* vol. 10 346. 7 Jun. 2019, doi:10.3389/fendo.2019.00346

Silvestris, Erica et al. "Obesity as disruptor of the female fertility." *Reproductive biology and endocrinology : RB&E* vol. 16,1 22. 9 Mar. 2018, doi:10.1186/s12958-018-0336-z

Simas, Joana N et al. "Resveratrol improves sperm DNA quality and reproductive capacity in type 1 diabetes." Andrology vol. 9,1 (2021): 384-399. doi:10.1111/andr.12891

Simopoulos, A P. "The importance of the ratio of omega-6/omega-3 essential fatty acids." *Biomedicine & pharmacotherapy = Biomedecine & pharmacotherapie* vol. 56,8 (2002): 365-79. doi:10.1016/s0753-3322(02)00253-6

Sirota, Ido et al. "Potential influence of the microbiome on infertility and assisted reproductive technology." *Seminars in reproductive medicine* vol. 32,1 (2014): 35-42. doi:10.1055/s-0033-1361821

Skoracka, Kinga et al. "Female Fertility and the Nutritional Approach: The Most Essential Aspects." *Advances in nutrition (Bethesda, Md.)* vol. 12,6 (2021): 2372-2386. doi:10.1093/advances/nmab068

Smits, Roos M et al. "Antioxidants for male subfertility." *The Cochrane database of systematic reviews* vol. 3,3 CD007411. 14 Mar. 2019, doi:10.1002/14651858.CD007411.pub4

Snider, Alexandria P, and Jennifer R Wood. "Obesity induces ovarian inflammation and reduces oocyte quality." *Reproduction (Cambridge, England)* vol. 158,3 (2019): R79-R90. doi:10.1530/REP-18-0583

Sortino, Maria A et al. "Polycystic Ovary Syndrome: Insights into the Therapeutic Approach with Inositols." Frontiers in pharmacology vol. 8 341. 8 Jun. 2017, doi:10.3389/fphar.2017.00341

Souter, I et al. "The association of protein intake (amount and type) with ovarian antral follicle counts among infertile women: results from the EARTH prospective study cohort." *BJOG : an international journal of obstetrics and gynaecology* vol. 124,10 (2017): 1547-1555. doi:10.1111/1471-0528.14630

Srivastava, Sudha et al. "Mechanism of action of L-arginine on the vitality of spermatozoa is primarily through increased biosynthesis of nitric oxide." Biology of reproduction vol. 74,5 (2006): 954-8. doi:10.1095/biolreprod.105.046896

Stanhiser, Jamie et al. "Serum omega-3 and omega-6 fatty acid concentrations and natural fertility." *Human reproduction (Oxford, England)* vol. 35,4 (2020): 950-957. doi:10.1093/humrep/dez305

Steegers-Theunissen, Régine et al. "Pre-Conception Interventions for Subfertile Couples Undergoing Assisted

Reproductive Technology Treatment: Modeling Analysis." JMIR mHealth and uHealth vol. 8,11 e19570. 23 Nov. 2020, doi:10.2196/19570

Stewart, D E et al. "Infertility and eating disorders." American journal of obstetrics and gynecology vol. 163,4 Pt 1 (1990): 1196-9. doi:10.1016/0002-9378(90)90688-4

Suleiman, S A et al. "Lipid peroxidation and human sperm motility: protective role of vitamin E." *Journal of andrology* vol. 17,5 (1996): 530-7.

Sun, Yangbo et al. "Association of Major Dietary Protein Sources With All-Cause and Cause-Specific Mortality: Prospective Cohort Study." *Journal of the American Heart Association* vol. 10,5 (2021): e015553. doi:10.1161/JAHA.119.015553

Swan, Shanna H. and Stacy Colino. Count Down: How Our Modern World Is Threatening Sperm Counts, Altering Male and Female Reproductive Development, and Imperiling the Future of the Human Race. Scribner, 2021.

Tachedjian, Gilda et al. "The implausible "in vivo" role of hydrogen peroxide as an antimicrobial factor produced by vaginal microbiota." *Microbiome* vol. 6,1 29. 6 Feb. 2018, doi:10.1186/s40168-018-0418-3

Taherian, Samira-Sadat et al. "Alpha-lipoic acid minimises reactive oxygen species-induced damages during sperm processing." *Andrologia* vol. 51,8 (2019): e13314. doi:10.1111/and.13314

Takasaki, Akihisa et al. "Endometrial growth and uterine blood flow: a pilot study for improving endometrial thickness in the patients with a thin endometrium." *Fertility and sterility* vol. 93,6 (2010): 1851-8. doi:10.1016/j.fertnstert.2008.12.062

Taş, Sibel et al. "Vitamin B6 supplementation improves oxidative stress and enhances serum paraoxonase/arylesterase activities in streptozotocin-induced diabetic rats." *TheScientificWorldJournal* vol. 2014 (2014): 351598. doi:10.1155/2014/351598

Thurston, Layla et al. "Investigation and management of subfertility." Journal of clinical pathology vol. 72,9 (2019): 579-587. doi:10.1136/jclinpath-2018-205579

Tiseo, Bruno C et al. "Coenzyme Q10 Intake From Food and Semen Parameters in a Subfertile Population." Urology vol. 102 (2017): 100-105. doi:10.1016/j.urology.2016.11.022

Tomaiuolo, Rossella et al. "Microbiota and Human Reproduction: The Case of Female Infertility." *High-throughput* vol. 9,2 12. 3 May. 2020, doi:10.3390/ht9020012

Tomaiuolo, Rossella et al. "Microbiota and Human Reproduction: The Case of Male Infertility." *High-throughput* vol. 9,2 10. 13 Apr. 2020, doi:10.3390/ht9020010

Torres-Arce, Elizabeth et al. "Dietary Antioxidants in the Treatment of Male Infertility: Counteracting Oxidative Stress." Biology vol. 10,3 241. 20 Mar. 2021, doi:10.3390/biology10030241

Tortoriello, Drew V et al. "Dietary-induced obesity and hypothalamic infertility in female DBA/2J mice." *Endocrinology* vol. 145,3 (2004): 1238-47. doi:10.1210/en.2003-1406

Toson, Bruno et al. "The Endometrial Microbiome and Its Impact on Human Conception." *International journal of molecular sciences* vol. 23,1 485. 1 Jan. 2022, doi:10.3390/ijms23010485

Tremellen, Kelton et al. "Metabolic endotoxaemia related inflammation is associated with hypogonadism in overweight men." *Basic and clinical andrology* vol. 27 5. 8 Mar. 2017, doi:10.1186/s12610-017-0049-8

Turnbaugh, Peter J et al. "The human microbiome project." *Nature* vol. 449,7164 (2007): 804-10. doi:10.1038/nature06244

Unfer, Vittorio et al. "Phytoestrogens may improve the pregnancy rate in in vitro fertilization-embryo transfer cycles: a prospective, controlled, randomized trial." *Fertility and sterility* vol. 82,6 (2004): 1509-13. doi:10.1016/j.fertnstert.2004.07.934

Valcarce, D G et al. "Probiotic administration improves sperm quality in asthenozoospermic human donors." *Beneficial microbes* vol. 8,2 (2017): 193-206. doi:10.3920/BM2016.0122

van de Lagemaat, Erik E et al. "Vitamin B_{12} in Relation to Oxidative Stress: A Systematic Review." *Nutrients* vol. 11,2 482. 25 Feb. 2019, doi:10.3390/nu11020482

van de Vijver, Arne et al. "Vitamin D deficiency and pregnancy rates following frozen-thawed embryo transfer: a prospective cohort study." *Human reproduction (Oxford, England)* vol. 31,8 (2016): 1749-54. doi:10.1093/humrep/dew107

van Oostrum, Noortje et al. "Risks associated with bacterial vaginosis in infertility patients: a systematic review and meta-analysis." *Human reproduction (Oxford, England)* vol. 28,7 (2013): 1809-15. doi:10.1093/humrep/det096

Vanegas, Jose C et al. "Soy food intake and treatment outcomes of women undergoing assisted reproductive technology." *Fertility and sterility* vol. 103,3 (2015): 749-55.e2. doi:10.1016/j.fertnstert.2014.12.104

Villegas, J et al. "Bacteria induce expression of apoptosis in human spermatozoa." *Apoptosis : an international journal on programmed cell death* vol. 10,1 (2005): 105-10. doi:10.1007/s10495-005-6065-8

Vitagliano, Amerigo et al. "Effects of chronic endometritis therapy on in vitro fertilization outcome in women with repeated implantation failure: a systematic review and meta-analysis." Fertility and sterility vol. 110,1 (2018): 103-112.e1. doi:10.1016/j.fertnstert.2018.03.017

Vujkovic, Marijana et al. "The preconception Mediterranean dietary pattern in couples undergoing in vitro fertilization/intracytoplasmic sperm injection treatment increases the chance of pregnancy." *Fertility and sterility* vol. 94,6 (2010): 2096-101. doi:10.1016/j.fertnstert.2009.12.079

Webb, Ann R et al. "Colour Counts: Sunlight and Skin Type as Drivers of Vitamin D Deficiency at UK Latitudes." *Nutrients* vol. 10,4 457. 7 Apr. 2018, doi:10.3390/nu10040457

Webb, Lauren. "Probiotics for preventing recurrent bacterial vaginosis." *JAAPA : official journal of the American Academy of Physician Assistants* vol. 34,2 (2021): 19-22. doi:10.1097/01.JAA.0000731484.81301.58

Wee, Bryan A et al. "A retrospective pilot study to determine whether the reproductive tract microbiota differs between women with a history of infertility and fertile women." *The Australian & New Zealand journal of obstetrics & gynaecology* vol. 58,3 (2018): 341-348. doi:10.1111/ajo.12754

Westphal, L M et al. "Double-blind, placebo-controlled study of Fertilityblend: a nutritional supplement for improving fertility in women." *Clinical and experimental obstetrics & gynecology* vol. 33,4 (2006): 205-8.

Westphal, Lynn M et al. "A nutritional supplement for improving fertility in women: a pilot study." *The Journal of reproductive medicine* vol. 49,4 (2004): 289-93.

Wiesenfeld, Harold C et al. "Bacterial vaginosis is a strong predictor of Neisseria gonorrhoeae and Chlamydia trachomatis infection." *Clinical infectious diseases : an official publication of the Infectious Diseases Society of America* vol. 36,5 (2003): 663-8. doi:10.1086/367658

Willis, Sydney K et al. "Glycemic load, dietary fiber, and added sugar and fecundability in 2 preconception cohorts." The

American journal of clinical nutrition vol. 112,1 (2020): 27-38. doi:10.1093/ajcn/nqz312

Wise, Lauren A et al. "Dairy intake and fecundability in 2 preconception cohort studies." *The American journal of clinical nutrition* vol. 105,1 (2017): 100-110. doi:10.3945/ajcn.116.138404

Wise, Lauren A et al. "Dietary Fat Intake and Fecundability in 2 Preconception Cohort Studies." *American journal of epidemiology* vol. 187,1 (2018): 60-74. doi:10.1093/aje/kwx204

Wong, Wai Yee et al. "Effects of folic acid and zinc sulfate on male factor subfertility: a double-blind, randomized, placebo-controlled trial." *Fertility and sterility* vol. 77,3 (2002): 491-8. doi:10.1016/s0015-0282(01)03229-0

Wu, Guoyao. "Dietary protein intake and human health." *Food & function* vol. 7,3 (2016): 1251-65. doi:10.1039/c5fo01530h

Xia, Wei et al. "Men's meat intake and treatment outcomes among couples undergoing assisted reproduction." Fertility and sterility vol. 104,4 (2015): 972-979. doi:10.1016/j.fertnstert.2015.06.037

Xue, Xia et al. "Cumulative Live Birth Rates According to Maternal Body Mass Index After First Ovarian Stimulation for in vitro Fertilization: A Single Center Analysis of 14,782 Patients." *Frontiers in endocrinology* vol. 11 149. 9 Apr. 2020, doi:10.3389/fendo.2020.00149

Yang, Qingling et al. "Effect of paternal overweight or obesity on IVF treatment outcomes and the possible mechanisms involved." *Scientific reports* vol. 6 29787. 14 Jul. 2016, doi:10.1038/srep29787

Yu, Shuai et al. "β-carotene improves oocyte development and maturation under oxidative stress in vitro." *In vitro cellular & developmental biology. Animal* vol. 55,7 (2019): 548-558. doi:10.1007/s11626-019-00373-0

Yuyan, Li et al. "Are serum zinc and copper levels related to semen quality?." *Fertility and sterility* vol. 89,4 (2008): 1008-11. doi:10.1016/j.fertnstert.2007.04.028

Zeisel, Steven H. "Epigenetic mechanisms for nutrition determinants of later health outcomes." The American journal of clinical nutrition vol. 89,5 (2009): 1488S-1493S. doi:10.3945/ajcn.2009.27113B

Zhao, Jiang et al. "Zinc levels in seminal plasma and their correlation with male infertility: A systematic review and meta-analysis." Scientific reports vol. 6 22386. 2 Mar. 2016, doi:10.1038/srep22386

Zheng, Xiangqin et al. "Inositol supplement improves clinical pregnancy rate in infertile women undergoing ovulation induction for ICSI or IVF-ET." *Medicine* vol. 96,49 (2017): e8842. doi:10.1097/MD.0000000000008842

Zhou, Xin et al. "Effect of L-carnitine and/or L-acetyl-carnitine in nutrition treatment for male infertility: a systematic review." Asia Pacific journal of clinical nutrition vol. 16 Suppl 1 (2007): 383-90.

About the Author

Clare Fleishman RDN, MS is a Registered Dietitian with the Academy of Nutrition and Dietetics and holds a master's degree in nutrition science. She bridges the gap between science and health across most platforms: major newspapers, magazines, books (Globesity), workshops, social media and websites. From corporate whiteboards to refugee schools in Egypt, Fleishman agitates for personal and public change. In 2010, she launched www.ProbioticsNow.com to share the cascade of new discoveries in the microbiome. Always amazed at this "forgotten organ" Fleishman also creates white papers, blogs, videos and social media for the International Probiotics Association as well as continuing education platforms.

End Notes

[1] https://www.nytimes.com/2021/11/20/style/breed-children-climate-change.html

[2] https://www.reproductivefacts.org/news-and-publications/patient-fact-sheets-and-booklets/documents/fact-sheets-and-info-booklets/age-and-fertility/

[3] https://www.cdc.gov/nchs/fastats/infertility.htm

[4] https://www.who.int/news-room/fact-sheets/detail/infertility

[5] Thurston, Layla et al. "Investigation and management of subfertility." Journal of clinical pathology vol. 72,9 (2019): 579-587. doi:10.1136/jclinpath-2018-205579

[6] Cariati, Federica et al. "The evolving role of genetic tests in reproductive medicine." Journal of translational medicine vol. 17,1 267. 14 Aug. 2019, doi:10.1186/s12967-019-2019-8

[7] Cariati, Federica et al. ""Bisphenol a: an emerging threat to male fertility"." Reproductive biology and endocrinology : RB&E vol. 17,1 6. 20 Jan. 2019, doi:10.1186/s12958-018-0447-6

[8] Bieniek, Jared M, and Kirk C Lo. "Recent advances in understanding & managing male infertility." F1000Research vol. 5 2756. 24 Nov. 2016, doi:10.12688/f1000research.9375.1

[9] Bieniek, Jared M, and Kirk C Lo. "Recent advances in understanding & managing male infertility." *F1000Research* vol. 5 2756. 24 Nov. 2016, doi:10.12688/f1000research.9375.1

[10] Rizzo, Anthony E et al. "The Female Reproductive Tract Microbiome-Implications for Gynecologic Cancers and Personalized Medicine." Journal of personalized medicine vol. 11,6 546. 11 Jun. 2021, doi:10.3390/jpm11060546

[11] Turnbaugh, Peter J et al. "The human microbiome project." Nature vol. 449,7164 (2007): 804-10. doi:10.1038/nature06244

[12] Moreno, Inmaculada, and Carlos Simon. "Deciphering the effect of reproductive tract microbiota on human reproduction." Reproductive medicine and biology vol. 18,1 40-50. 1 Nov. 2018, doi:10.1002/rmb2.12249

---

[13] Tomaiuolo, Rossella et al. "Microbiota and Human Reproduction: The Case of Female Infertility." *High-throughput* vol. 9,2 12. 3 May. 2020, doi:10.3390/ht9020012

[14] Moreno, Inmaculada, and Jason M Franasiak. "Endometrial microbiota-new player in town." Fertility and sterility vol. 108,1 (2017): 32-39. doi:10.1016/j.fertnstert.2017.05.034

[15] Fernández, Leónides et al. "Application of Ligilactobacillus salivarius CECT5713 to Achieve Term Pregnancies in Women with Repetitive Abortion or Infertility of Unknown Origin by Microbiological and Immunological Modulation of the Vaginal Ecosystem." Nutrients vol. 13,1 162. 6 Jan. 2021, doi:10.3390/nu13010162

[16] Moreno, Inmaculada, and Carlos Simon. "Deciphering the effect of reproductive tract microbiota on human reproduction." Reproductive medicine and biology vol. 18,1 40-50. 1 Nov. 2018, doi:10.1002/rmb2.12249

[17] D'Argenio, Valeria. "The Prenatal Microbiome: A New Player for Human Health." High-throughput vol. 7,4 38. 11 Dec. 2018, doi:10.3390/ht7040038

[18] Chen, Chen et al. "The microbiota continuum along the female reproductive tract and its relation to uterine-related diseases." Nature communications vol. 8,1 875. 17 Oct. 2017, doi:10.1038/s41467-017-00901-0

[19] Benner, Marilen et al. "How uterine microbiota might be responsible for a receptive, fertile endometrium." Human reproduction update vol. 24,4 (2018): 393-415. doi:10.1093/humupd/dmy012

[20] Moreno, Inmaculada et al. "Evidence that the endometrial microbiota has an effect on implantation success or failure." American journal of obstetrics and gynecology vol. 215,6 (2016): 684-703. doi:10.1016/j.ajog.2016.09.075

[21] Tomaiuolo, Rossella et al. "Microbiota and Human Reproduction: The Case of Female Infertility." High-throughput vol. 9,2 12. 3 May. 2020, doi:10.3390/ht9020012

[22] Tomaiuolo, Rossella et al. "Microbiota and Human Reproduction: The Case of Female Infertility." High-throughput vol. 9,2 12. 3 May. 2020, doi:10.3390/ht9020012

[23] Younis, N., Mahasneh, A. Probiotics and the envisaged role in treating human infertility. Middle East Fertil Soc J 25, 33 (2020). https://doi.org/10.1186/s43043-020-00039-y

[24] Delaney, M L, and A B Onderdonk. "Nugent score related to vaginal culture in pregnant women." Obstetrics and gynecology vol. 98,1 (2001): 79-84. doi:10.1016/s0029-7844(01)01402-8

[25] Ravel, Jacques et al. "Vaginal microbiome of reproductive-age women." Proceedings of the National Academy of Sciences of the United States of America vol. 108 Suppl 1,Suppl 1 (2011): 4680-7. doi:10.1073/pnas.1002611107

[26] Ravel, Jacques et al. "Vaginal microbiome of reproductive-age women." Proceedings of the National Academy of Sciences of the United States of America vol. 108 Suppl 1,Suppl 1 (2011): 4680-7. doi:10.1073/pnas.1002611107

[27] Bradshaw, Catriona S et al. "Prevalent and incident bacterial vaginosis are associated with sexual and contraceptive behaviours in young Australian women." PloS one vol. 8,3 (2013): e57688. doi:10.1371/journal.pone.0057688

[28] Anahtar, Melis N et al. "Cervicovaginal Microbiota and Reproductive Health: The Virtue of Simplicity." Cell host & microbe vol. 23,2 (2018): 159-168. doi:10.1016/j.chom.2018.01.013

[29] Anahtar, Melis N et al. "Cervicovaginal Microbiota and Reproductive Health: The Virtue of Simplicity." Cell host & microbe vol. 23,2 (2018): 159-168. doi:10.1016/j.chom.2018.01.013

[30] Aldunate, Muriel et al. "Antimicrobial and immune modulatory effects of lactic acid and short chain fatty acids produced by vaginal microbiota associated with eubiosis and bacterial vaginosis." Frontiers in physiology vol. 6 164. 2 Jun. 2015, doi:10.3389/fphys.2015.00164

[31] Tachedjian, Gilda et al. "The implausible "in vivo" role of hydrogen peroxide as an antimicrobial factor produced by vaginal microbiota." Microbiome vol. 6,1 29. 6 Feb. 2018, doi:10.1186/s40168-018-0418-3

[32] Moreno, Inmaculada, and Carlos Simon. "Deciphering the effect of reproductive tract microbiota on human reproduction." Reproductive medicine and biology vol. 18,1 40-50. 1 Nov. 2018, doi:10.1002/rmb2.12249

[33] Aldunate, Muriel et al. "Antimicrobial and immune modulatory effects of lactic acid and short chain fatty acids produced by vaginal microbiota associated with eubiosis and bacterial vaginosis." Frontiers in physiology vol. 6 164. 2 Jun. 2015, doi:10.3389/fphys.2015.00164

[34] Noyes, Noelle et al. "Associations between sexual habits, menstrual hygiene practices, demographics and the vaginal microbiome as revealed by Bayesian network analysis." PloS one vol. 13,1 e0191625. 24 Jan. 2018, doi:10.1371/journal.pone.0191625

[35] https://www.ncbi.nlm.nih.gov/pmc/articles/PMC6332752/figure/rmb212249-fig-0001/

[36] Peebles, Kathryn et al. "High Global Burden and Costs of Bacterial Vaginosis: A Systematic Review and Meta-Analysis." Sexually transmitted diseases vol. 46,5 (2019): 304-311. doi:10.1097/OLQ.0000000000000972

[37] Bagnall, Paulette, and Denise Rizzolo. "Bacterial vaginosis: A practical review." JAAPA : official journal of the American Academy of Physician Assistants vol. 30,12 (2017): 15-21. doi:10.1097/01.JAA.0000526770.60197.fa

[38] Powell, Anna et al. "Clinicians' Use of Intravaginal Boric Acid Maintenance Therapy for Recurrent Vulvovaginal Candidiasis and Bacterial Vaginosis." Sexually transmitted diseases vol. 46,12 (2019): 810-812. doi:10.1097/OLQ.0000000000001063

[39] Fredricks, David N et al. "Molecular identification of bacteria associated with bacterial vaginosis." The New England journal of medicine vol. 353,18 (2005): 1899-911. doi:10.1056/NEJMoa043802

[40] Rizzo, Anthony E et al. "The Female Reproductive Tract Microbiome-Implications for Gynecologic Cancers and Personalized Medicine." Journal of personalized medicine vol. 11,6 546. 11 Jun. 2021, doi:10.3390/jpm11060546

[41] Mendling W. (2016) Vaginal Microbiota. In: Schwiertz A. (eds) Microbiota of the Human Body. Advances in Experimental Medicine and Biology, vol 902. Springer, Cham. https://doi.org/10.1007/978-3-319-31248-4_6

[42] Juárez Tomás, María Silvina et al. "Growth and lactic acid production by vaginal Lactobacillus acidophilus CRL 1259, and inhibition of uropathogenic Escherichia coli." Journal of medical microbiology vol. 52,Pt 12 (2003): 1117-1124. doi:10.1099/jmm.0.05155-0

[43] Wiggins, R et al. "Mucinases and sialidases: their role in the pathogenesis of sexually transmitted infections in the female genital tract." Sexually transmitted infections vol. 77,6 (2001): 402-8. doi:10.1136/sti.77.6.402

[44] Harwich, Michael D Jr et al. "Drawing the line between commensal and pathogenic Gardnerella vaginalis through genome analysis and virulence

studies." BMC genomics vol. 11 375. 11 Jun. 2010, doi:10.1186/1471-2164-11-375

[45] Fernández, Leónides et al. "Application of Ligilactobacillus salivarius CECT5713 to Achieve Term Pregnancies in Women with Repetitive Abortion or Infertility of Unknown Origin by Microbiological and Immunological Modulation of the Vaginal Ecosystem." Nutrients vol. 13,1 162. 6 Jan. 2021, doi:10.3390/nu13010162

[46] van Oostrum, Noortje et al. "Risks associated with bacterial vaginosis in infertility patients: a systematic review and meta-analysis." Human reproduction (Oxford, England) vol. 28,7 (2013): 1809-15. doi:10.1093/humrep/det096

[47] Fernández, Leónides et al. "Application of Ligilactobacillus salivarius CECT5713 to Achieve Term Pregnancies in Women with Repetitive Abortion or Infertility of Unknown Origin by Microbiological and Immunological Modulation of the Vaginal Ecosystem." Nutrients vol. 13,1 162. 6 Jan. 2021, doi:10.3390/nu13010162

[48] Ravel, Jacques et al. "Bacterial vaginosis and its association with infertility, endometritis, and pelvic inflammatory disease." *American journal of obstetrics and gynecology* vol. 224,3 (2021): 251-257. doi:10.1016/j.ajog.2020.10.019

[49] Kroon, Samuel J et al. "Cervicovaginal microbiota, women's health, and reproductive outcomes." Fertility and sterility vol. 110,3 (2018): 327-336. doi:10.1016/j.fertnstert.2018.06.036

[50] Bohbot, J M et al. "Efficacy and safety of vaginally administered lyophilized Lactobacillus crispatus IP 174178 in the prevention of bacterial vaginosis recurrence." Journal of gynecology obstetrics and human reproduction vol. 47,2 (2018): 81-86. doi:10.1016/j.jogoh.2017.11.005

[51] Moreno, Inmaculada et al. "The diagnosis of chronic endometritis in infertile asymptomatic women: a comparative study of histology, microbial cultures, hysteroscopy, and molecular microbiology." American journal of obstetrics and gynecology vol. 218,6 (2018): 602.e1-602.e16. doi:10.1016/j.ajog.2018.02.012

[52] Moreno, Inmaculada, and Jason M Franasiak. "Endometrial microbiota-new player in town." Fertility and sterility vol. 108,1 (2017): 32-39. doi:10.1016/j.fertnstert.2017.05.034

[53] López-Moreno, Ana, and Margarita Aguilera. "Probiotics Dietary Supplementation for Modulating Endocrine and Fertility Microbiota Dysbiosis." Nutrients vol. 12,3 757. 13 Mar. 2020, doi:10.3390/nu12030757

[54] Toson, Bruno et al. "The Endometrial Microbiome and Its Impact on Human Conception." *International journal of molecular sciences* vol. 23,1 485. 1 Jan. 2022, doi:10.3390/ijms23010485

[55] Moreno, Inmaculada et al. "Endometrial microbiota composition is associated with reproductive outcome in infertile patients." *Microbiome* vol. 10,1 1. 4 Jan. 2022, doi:10.1186/s40168-021-01184-w

[56] Sharma, Harsha et al. "Microbiota and pelvic inflammatory disease." Seminars in reproductive medicine vol. 32,1 (2014): 43-9. doi:10.1055/s-0033-1361822

[57] Hosseinzadeh, Pardis et al. "Polycystic Ovary Syndrome and the Forgotten Uterus." F&S reviews vol. 2,1 (2021): 11-20. doi:10.1016/j.xfnr.2020.12.001

[58] Cariati, Federica et al. "The evolving role of genetic tests in reproductive medicine." Journal of translational medicine vol. 17,1 267. 14 Aug. 2019, doi:10.1186/s12967-019-2019-8

[59] Tomaiuolo, Rossella et al. "Microbiota and Human Reproduction: The Case of Female Infertility." High-throughput vol. 9,2 12. 3 May. 2020, doi:10.3390/ht9020012

[60] Swan, Shanna H. and Stacy Colino. Count Down: How Our Modern World Is Threatening Sperm Counts, Altering Male and Female Reproductive Development, and Imperiling the Future of the Human Race. Scribner, 2021.

[61] https://marinfertilitycenter.com/new-getting-started/infertility-basics/

[62] Tomaiuolo, Rossella et al. "Microbiota and Human Reproduction: The Case of Female Infertility." High-throughput vol. 9,2 12. 3 May. 2020, doi:10.3390/ht9020012

[63] Wee, Bryan A et al. "A retrospective pilot study to determine whether the reproductive tract microbiota differs between women with a history of infertility and fertile women." The Australian & New Zealand journal of obstetrics & gynaecology vol. 58,3 (2018): 341-348. doi:10.1111/ajo.12754

[64] Campisciano, Giuseppina et al. "Subclinical alteration of the cervical-vaginal microbiome in women with idiopathic infertility." Journal of cellular physiology vol. 232,7 (2017): 1681-1688. doi:10.1002/jcp.25806

[65] Hyman, Richard W et al. "The dynamics of the vaginal microbiome during infertility therapy with in vitro fertilization-embryo transfer." Journal of assisted reproduction and genetics vol. 29,2 (2012): 105-15. doi:10.1007/s10815-011-9694-6

[66] Haahr, T et al. "Abnormal vaginal microbiota may be associated with poor reproductive outcomes: a prospective study in IVF patients." Human reproduction (Oxford, England) vol. 31,4 (2016): 795-803. doi:10.1093/humrep/dew026

[67] Kyono, Koichi et al. "Analysis of endometrial microbiota by 16S ribosomal RNA gene sequencing among infertile patients: a single-center pilot study." Reproductive medicine and biology vol. 17,3 297-306. 6 May. 2018, doi:10.1002/rmb2.12105

[68] Garcia-Grau, Iolanda et al. "Taxonomical and Functional Assessment of the Endometrial Microbiota in A Context of Recurrent Reproductive Failure: A Case Report." Pathogens (Basel, Switzerland) vol. 8,4 205. 24 Oct. 2019, doi:10.3390/pathogens8040205

[69] Moreno, Inmaculada et al. "Evidence that the endometrial microbiota has an effect on implantation success or failure." American journal of obstetrics and gynecology vol. 215,6 (2016): 684-703. doi:10.1016/j.ajog.2016.09.075

[70] Hashimoto, Tomoko, and Koichi Kyono. "Does dysbiotic endometrium affect blastocyst implantation in IVF patients?." Journal of assisted reproduction and genetics vol. 36,12 (2019): 2471-2479. doi:10.1007/s10815-019-01630-7

[71] Sirota, Ido et al. "Potential influence of the microbiome on infertility and assisted reproductive technology." Seminars in reproductive medicine vol. 32,1 (2014): 35-42. doi:10.1055/s-0033-1361821

[72] Egbase, P E et al. "Incidence of microbial growth from the tip of the embryo transfer catheter after embryo transfer in relation to clinical pregnancy rate following in-vitro fertilization and embryo transfer." Human reproduction (Oxford, England) vol. 11,8 (1996): 1687-9. doi:10.1093/oxfordjournals.humrep.a019470

[73] Moreno, Inmaculada, and Carlos Simon. "Deciphering the effect of reproductive tract microbiota on human reproduction." Reproductive medicine and biology vol. 18,1 40-50. 1 Nov. 2018, doi:10.1002/rmb2.12249

[74] Cicinelli, Ettore et al. "Chronic endometritis in patients with unexplained infertility: Prevalence and effects of antibiotic treatment on spontaneous conception." American journal of reproductive immunology (New York, N.Y. : 1989) vol. 79,1 (2018): 10.1111/aji.12782. doi:10.1111/aji.12782

[75] Cicinelli, Ettore et al. "Chronic endometritis due to common bacteria is prevalent in women with recurrent miscarriage as confirmed by improved pregnancy outcome after antibiotic treatment." Reproductive sciences (Thousand Oaks, Calif.) vol. 21,5 (2014): 640-7. doi:10.1177/1933719113508817

[76] Vitagliano, Amerigo et al. "Effects of chronic endometritis therapy on in vitro fertilization outcome in women with repeated implantation failure: a systematic review and meta-analysis." Fertility and sterility vol. 110,1 (2018): 103-112.e1. doi:10.1016/j.fertnstert.2018.03.017

[77] Hill, Colin et al. "Expert consensus document. The International Scientific Association for Probiotics and Prebiotics consensus statement on the scope and appropriate use of the term probiotic." Nature reviews. Gastroenterology & hepatology vol. 11,8 (2014): 506-14. doi:10.1038/nrgastro.2014.66

[78] Tomaiuolo, Rossella et al. "Microbiota and Human Reproduction: The Case of Female Infertility." High-throughput vol. 9,2 12. 3 May. 2020, doi:10.3390/ht9020012

[79] Anukam, Kingsley C et al. "Clinical study comparing probiotic Lactobacillus GR-1 and RC-14 with metronidazole vaginal gel to treat symptomatic bacterial vaginosis." Microbes and infection vol. 8,12-13 (2006): 2772-6. doi:10.1016/j.micinf.2006.08.008

[80] Mastromarino, P et al. "Effectiveness of Lactobacillus-containing vaginal tablets in the treatment of symptomatic bacterial vaginosis." Clinical microbiology and infection : the official publication of the European Society of Clinical Microbiology and Infectious Diseases vol. 15,1 (2009): 67-74. doi:10.1111/j.1469-0691.2008.02112.x

[81] López-Moreno, Ana, and Margarita Aguilera. "Vaginal Probiotics for Reproductive Health and Related Dysbiosis: Systematic Review and Meta-Analysis." Journal of clinical medicine vol. 10,7 1461. 2 Apr. 2021, doi:10.3390/jcm10071461

[82] Lagenaur, Laurel A et al. "Connecting the Dots: Translating the Vaginal Microbiome Into a Drug." The Journal of infectious diseases vol. 223,12 Suppl 2 (2021): S296-S306. doi:10.1093/infdis/jiaa676

[83] Ling, Zongxin et al. "The restoration of the vaginal microbiota after treatment for bacterial vaginosis with metronidazole or probiotics." Microbial ecology vol. 65,3 (2013): 773-80. doi:10.1007/s00248-012-0154-3

[84] Recine, Nadia et al. "Restoring vaginal microbiota: biological control of bacterial vaginosis. A prospective case-control study using Lactobacillus rhamnosus BMX 54 as adjuvant treatment against bacterial vaginosis." Archives of gynecology and obstetrics vol. 293,1 (2016): 101-107. doi:10.1007/s00404-015-3810-2

[85] Petrova, Mariya I et al. "Lacticaseibacillus rhamnosus GR-1, a.k.a. Lactobacillus rhamnosus GR-1: Past and Future Perspectives." *Trends in microbiology* vol. 29,8 (2021): 747-761. doi:10.1016/j.tim.2021.03.010

[86] López-Moreno, Ana, and Margarita Aguilera. "Vaginal Probiotics for Reproductive Health and Related Dysbiosis: Systematic Review and Meta-Analysis." *Journal of clinical medicine* vol. 10,7 1461. 2 Apr. 2021, doi:10.3390/jcm10071461

[87] Bradshaw, Catriona S et al. "High recurrence rates of bacterial vaginosis over the course of 12 months after oral metronidazole therapy and factors associated with recurrence." *The Journal of infectious diseases* vol. 193,11 (2006): 1478-86. doi:10.1086/503780

[88] Moreno, Inmaculada, and Carlos Simon. "Deciphering the effect of reproductive tract microbiota on human reproduction." Reproductive medicine and biology vol. 18,1 40-50. 1 Nov. 2018, doi:10.1002/rmb2.12249

[89] Tomaiuolo, Rossella et al. "Microbiota and Human Reproduction: The Case of Female Infertility." High-throughput vol. 9,2 12. 3 May. 2020, doi:10.3390/ht9020012

[90] Moreno, Inmaculada, and Carlos Simon. "Deciphering the effect of reproductive tract microbiota on human reproduction." Reproductive medicine and biology vol. 18,1 40-50. 1 Nov. 2018, doi:10.1002/rmb2.12249

[91] Corbett, G A et al. "Probiotic therapy in couples with infertility: A systematic review." European journal of obstetrics, gynecology, and reproductive biology vol. 256 (2021): 95-100. doi:10.1016/j.ejogrb.2020.10.054

[92] Ohri, Manju, and Vijay Prabha. "Isolation of a sperm-agglutinating factor from Staphylococcus aureus isolated from a woman with unexplained infertility." Fertility and sterility vol. 84,5 (2005): 1539-41. doi:10.1016/j.fertnstert.2005.05.030

[93] Fernández, Leónides et al. "Application of Ligilactobacillus salivarius CECT5713 to Achieve Term Pregnancies in Women with Repetitive Abortion or Infertility of Unknown Origin by Microbiological and Immunological Modulation of the Vaginal Ecosystem." Nutrients vol. 13,1 162. 6 Jan. 2021, doi:10.3390/nu13010162

[94]Ghanei, Nila et al. "The probiotic supplementation reduced inflammation in polycystic ovary syndrome: A randomized, double-blind, placebo-controlled trial."Journal of Functional Foods vol 42 (2018): 306-311, doi.org/10.1016/j.jff.2017.12.047.

[95] Gibson, Glenn R et al. "Expert consensus document: The International Scientific Association for Probiotics and Prebiotics (ISAPP) consensus statement on the definition and scope of prebiotics." *Nature reviews. Gastroenterology & hepatology* vol. 14,8 (2017): 491-502. doi:10.1038/nrgastro.2017.75

[96] Komiya, Shinnosuke et al. "Characterizing the gut microbiota in females with infertility and preliminary results of a water-soluble dietary fiber intervention study." *Journal of clinical biochemistry and nutrition* vol. 67,1 (2020): 105-111. doi:10.3164/jcbn.20-53

[97] Altmäe, Signe. "Commentary: Uterine Microbiota: Residents, Tourists, or Invaders?." Frontiers in immunology vol. 9 1874. 24 Aug. 2018, doi:10.3389/fimmu.2018.01874

[98] Plummer, Erica L et al. "Combined oral and topical antimicrobial therapy for male partners of women with bacterial vaginosis: Acceptability, tolerability and impact on the genital microbiota of couples - A pilot study." PloS one vol. 13,1 e0190199. 2 Jan. 2018, doi:10.1371/journal.pone.0190199

[99] Moreno, Inmaculada, and Carlos Simon. "Deciphering the effect of reproductive tract microbiota on human reproduction." Reproductive medicine and biology vol. 18,1 40-50. 1 Nov. 2018, doi:10.1002/rmb2.12249

[100] Mändar, Reet et al. "Complementary seminovaginal microbiome in couples." Research in microbiology vol. 166,5 (2015): 440-447. doi:10.1016/j.resmic.2015.03.009

[101] Hales, Craig M et al. "Prevalence of Obesity and Severe Obesity Among Adults: United States, 2017-2018." NCHS data brief ,360 (2020): 1-8.

[102] Silvestris, Erica et al. "Obesity as disruptor of the female fertility." *Reproductive biology and endocrinology : RB&E* vol. 16,1 22. 9 Mar. 2018, doi:10.1186/s12958-018-0336-z

[103] Broughton, Darcy E, and Kelle H Moley. "Obesity and female infertility: potential mediators of obesity's impact." Fertility and sterility vol. 107,4 (2017): 840-847. doi:10.1016/j.fertnstert.2017.01.017

[104] Mikhael, Sasha et al. "Hypothalamic-Pituitary-Ovarian Axis Disorders Impacting Female Fertility." Biomedicines vol. 7,1 5. 4 Jan. 2019, doi:10.3390/biomedicines7010005

[105] Tortoriello, Drew V et al. "Dietary-induced obesity and hypothalamic infertility in female DBA/2J mice." Endocrinology vol. 145,3 (2004): 1238-47. doi:10.1210/en.2003-1406

[106] Jain, Akas et al. "Pulsatile luteinizing hormone amplitude and progesterone metabolite excretion are reduced in obese women." The Journal of clinical endocrinology and metabolism vol. 92,7 (2007): 2468-73. doi:10.1210/jc.2006-2274

[107] Broughton, Darcy E, and Kelle H Moley. "Obesity and female infertility: potential mediators of obesity's impact." *Fertility and sterility* vol. 107,4 (2017): 840-847. doi:10.1016/j.fertnstert.2017.01.017

[108] Leary, Christine et al. "Human embryos from overweight and obese women display phenotypic and metabolic abnormalities." Human reproduction (Oxford, England) vol. 30,1 (2015): 122-32. doi:10.1093/humrep/deu276

[109] Snider, Alexandria P, and Jennifer R Wood. "Obesity induces ovarian inflammation and reduces oocyte quality." *Reproduction (Cambridge, England)* vol. 158,3 (2019): R79-R90. doi:10.1530/REP-18-0583

[110] Silvestris, Erica et al. "Obesity as disruptor of the female fertility." *Reproductive biology and endocrinology : RB&E* vol. 16,1 22. 9 Mar. 2018, doi:10.1186/s12958-018-0336-z

[111] Silvestris, Erica et al. "Obesity as disruptor of the female fertility." Reproductive biology and endocrinology : RB&E vol. 16,1 22. 9 Mar. 2018, doi:10.1186/s12958-018-0336-z

[112] Okada, Hidetaka et al. "Decidualization of the human endometrium." Reproductive medicine and biology vol. 17,3 220-227. 1 Feb. 2018, doi:10.1002/rmb2.12088

[113] Hohos, Natalie M, and Malgorzata E Skaznik-Wikiel. "High-Fat Diet and Female Fertility." Endocrinology vol. 158,8 (2017): 2407-2419. doi:10.1210/en.2017-00371

[114] Sarais, Veronica et al. "A Comprehensive Analysis of Body Mass Index Effect on in Vitro Fertilization Outcomes." Nutrients vol. 8,3 109. 23 Feb. 2016, doi:10.3390/nu8030109

[115] Robker, Rebecca L et al. "Obese women exhibit differences in ovarian metabolites, hormones, and gene expression compared with moderate-weight women." The Journal of clinical endocrinology and metabolism vol. 94,5 (2009): 1533-40. doi:10.1210/jc.2008-2648

[116] Broughton, Darcy E, and Kelle H Moley. "Obesity and female infertility: potential mediators of obesity's impact." Fertility and sterility vol. 107,4 (2017): 840-847. doi:10.1016/j.fertnstert.2017.01.017

[117] Xue, Xia et al. "Cumulative Live Birth Rates According to Maternal Body Mass Index After First Ovarian Stimulation for in vitro Fertilization: A Single Center Analysis of 14,782 Patients." Frontiers in endocrinology vol. 11 149. 9 Apr. 2020, doi:10.3389/fendo.2020.00149

[118] WHO Expert Consultation. "Appropriate body-mass index for Asian populations and its implications for policy and intervention strategies." Lancet (London, England) vol. 363,9403 (2004): 157-63. doi:10.1016/S0140-6736(03)15268-3

[119] Gaskins, Audrey J et al. "Substantial Weight Gain in Adulthood Is Associated with Lower Probability of Live Birth Following Assisted Reproduction." The Journal of nutrition vol. 151,3 (2021): 649-656. doi:10.1093/jn/nxaa371

[120] Mutsaerts, Meike A Q et al. "Randomized Trial of a Lifestyle Program in Obese Infertile Women." The New England journal of medicine vol. 374,20 (2016): 1942-53. doi:10.1056/NEJMoa1505297

[121] Chavarro, Jorge E et al. "Body mass index and short-term weight change in relation to treatment outcomes in women undergoing assisted reproduction." Fertility and sterility vol. 98,1 (2012): 109-16. doi:10.1016/j.fertnstert.2012.04.012

---

[122] Broughton, Darcy E, and Kelle H Moley. "Obesity and female infertility: potential mediators of obesity's impact." Fertility and sterility vol. 107,4 (2017): 840-847. doi:10.1016/j.fertnstert.2017.01.017

[123] Steegers-Theunissen, Régine et al. "Pre-Conception Interventions for Subfertile Couples Undergoing Assisted Reproductive Technology Treatment: Modeling Analysis." JMIR mHealth and uHealth vol. 8,11 e19570. 23 Nov. 2020, doi:10.2196/19570

[124] Best, Damian et al. "How effective are weight-loss interventions for improving fertility in women and men who are overweight or obese? A systematic review and meta-analysis of the evidence." Human reproduction update vol. 23,6 (2017): 681-705. doi:10.1093/humupd/dmx027

[125] Palomba, Stefano et al. "Physical activity before IVF and ICSI cycles in infertile obese women: an observational cohort study." Reproductive biomedicine online vol. 29,1 (2014): 72-9. doi:10.1016/j.rbmo.2014.03.006

[126] Farinha, Juliano Boufleur et al. "Response of oxidative stress and inflammatory biomarkers to a 12-week aerobic exercise training in women with metabolic syndrome." Sports medicine - open vol. 1,1 (2015): 19. doi:10.1186/s40798-015-0011-2

[127] Biviá-Roig, Gemma et al. "Impact of the COVID-19 Pandemic on the Lifestyles and Quality of Life of Women With Fertility Problems: A Cross-Sectional Study." Frontiers in public health vol. 9 686115. 19 Jul. 2021, doi:10.3389/fpubh.2021.686115

[128] Johansson, Kari et al. "Outcomes of pregnancy after bariatric surgery." The New England journal of medicine vol. 372,9 (2015): 814-24. doi:10.1056/NEJMoa1405789

[129] Escobar-Morreale, Héctor F et al. "The polycystic ovary syndrome associated with morbid obesity may resolve after weight loss induced by bariatric surgery." The Journal of clinical endocrinology and metabolism vol. 90,12 (2005): 6364-9. doi:10.1210/jc.2005-1490

[130] Chang, Catherine et al. "The Impact of Bariatric Surgery Compared to Metformin Therapy on Pregnancy Outcomes in Patients with Polycystic Ovarian Syndrome: a Systematic Review and Meta-analysis." Journal of gastrointestinal surgery : official journal of the Society for Surgery of the Alimentary Tract vol. 25,2 (2021): 378-386. doi:10.1007/s11605-020-04900-3

[131] Silvestris, Erica et al. "Obesity as disruptor of the female fertility." Reproductive biology and endocrinology : RB&E vol. 16,1 22. 9 Mar. 2018, doi:10.1186/s12958-018-0336-z

[132] Imterat, Majdi et al. "Impact of Body Mass Index on female fertility and ART outcomes." Panminerva medica vol. 61,1 (2019): 58-67. doi:10.23736/S0031-0808.18.03490-0

[133] Hashan, Mohammad Rashidul et al. "Prevalence and associated factors of underweight, overweight and obesity among women of reproductive age group in the Maldives: Evidence from a nationally representative study." *PloS one* vol. 15,10 e0241621. 29 Oct. 2020, doi:10.1371/journal.pone.0241621

[134] Boutari, Chrysoula et al. "The effect of underweight on female and male reproduction." Metabolism: clinical and experimental vol. 107 (2020): 154229. doi:10.1016/j.metabol.2020.154229

[135] Grodstein, F et al. "Body mass index and ovulatory infertility." Epidemiology (Cambridge, Mass.) vol. 5,2 (1994): 247-50. doi:10.1097/00001648-199403000-00016

[136] Han, Zhen et al. "Maternal underweight and the risk of preterm birth and low birth weight: a systematic review and meta-analyses." International journal of epidemiology vol. 40,1 (2011): 65-101. doi:10.1093/ije/dyq195

[137] Qian, Jie et al. "An update on the prevalence of eating disorders in the general population: a systematic review and meta-analysis." Eating and weight disorders : EWD, 10.1007/s40519-021-01162-z. 8 Apr. 2021, doi:10.1007/s40519-021-01162-z

[138] Bulik, C M et al. "Fertility and reproduction in women with anorexia nervosa: a controlled study." The Journal of clinical psychiatry vol. 60,2 (1999): 130-5; quiz 135-7. doi:10.4088/jcp.v60n0212

[139] Hecht, Leah M et al. "Disordered eating and eating disorders among women seeking fertility treatment: A systematic review." Archives of women's mental health, 10.1007/s00737-021-01156-x. 27 Jun. 2021, doi:10.1007/s00737-021-01156-x

[140] Kimmel, M C et al. "Obstetric and gynecologic problems associated with eating disorders." The International journal of eating disorders vol. 49,3 (2016): 260-75. doi:10.1002/eat.22483

[141] Mason, Helen D et al. "Pelvic ultrasonography in anorexia nervosa: what the clinician should ask the radiologist and how to use the information

provided." European eating disorders review : the journal of the Eating Disorders Association vol. 15,1 (2007): 35-41. doi:10.1002/erv.719

[142] Stewart, D E et al. "Infertility and eating disorders." American journal of obstetrics and gynecology vol. 163,4 Pt 1 (1990): 1196-9. doi:10.1016/0002-9378(90)90688-4

[143] Chaer, Rayane et al. "Fertility and Reproduction after Recovery from Anorexia Nervosa: A Systematic Review and Meta-Analysis of Long-Term Follow-Up Studies." Diseases (Basel, Switzerland) vol. 8,4 46. 16 Dec. 2020, doi:10.3390/diseases8040046

[144] Hoffman, Elizabeth R et al. "Reproductive issues in anorexia nervosa." Expert review of obstetrics & gynecology vol. 6,4 (2011): 403-414. doi:10.1586/eog.11.31

[145] Janas-Kozik, Małgorzata et al. "Systematic Review of Literature on Eating Disorders During Pregnancy-Risk and Consequences for Mother and Child." *Frontiers in psychiatry* vol. 12 777529. 13 Dec. 2021, doi:10.3389/fpsyt.2021.777529

[146] Zeisel, Steven H. "Epigenetic mechanisms for nutrition determinants of later health outcomes." The American journal of clinical nutrition vol. 89,5 (2009): 1488S-1493S. doi:10.3945/ajcn.2009.27113B

[147] Schlotz, Wolff, and David I W Phillips. "Fetal origins of mental health: evidence and mechanisms." Brain, behavior, and immunity vol. 23,7 (2009): 905-16. doi:10.1016/j.bbi.2009.02.001

[148] Gluckman, Peter D, and Mark A Hanson. "Living with the past: evolution, development, and patterns of disease." Science (New York, N.Y.) vol. 305,5691 (2004): 1733-6. doi:10.1126/science.1095292

[149] Zeisel, Steven H. "Epigenetic mechanisms for nutrition determinants of later health outcomes." The American journal of clinical nutrition vol. 89,5 (2009): 1488S-1493S. doi:10.3945/ajcn.2009.27113B

[150] Schlotz, Wolff, and David I W Phillips. "Fetal origins of mental health: evidence and mechanisms." Brain, behavior, and immunity vol. 23,7 (2009): 905-16. doi:10.1016/j.bbi.2009.02.001

[151] Seckl, Jonathan R, and Megan C Holmes. "Mechanisms of disease: glucocorticoids, their placental metabolism and fetal 'programming' of adult pathophysiology." Nature clinical practice. Endocrinology & metabolism vol. 3,6 (2007): 479-88. doi:10.1038/ncpendmet0515

[152] Hoffman, Elizabeth R et al. "Reproductive issues in anorexia nervosa." Expert review of obstetrics & gynecology vol. 6,4 (2011): 403-414. doi:10.1586/eog.11.31

[153] Jodar, Meritxell et al. "The protein and transcript profiles of human semen." Cell and tissue research vol. 363,1 (2016): 85-96. doi:10.1007/s00441-015-2237-1

[154] Palmer, Nicole O et al. "Impact of obesity on male fertility, sperm function and molecular composition." Spermatogenesis vol. 2,4 (2012): 253-263. doi:10.4161/spmg.21362

[155] Eisenberg, Michael L et al. "Increased risk of incident chronic medical conditions in infertile men: analysis of United States claims data." Fertility and sterility vol. 105,3 (2016): 629-636. doi:10.1016/j.fertnstert.2015.11.011

[156] Cavallini, Giorgio. "Male idiopathic oligoasthenoteratozoospermia." Asian journal of andrology vol. 8,2 (2006): 143-57. doi:10.1111/j.1745-7262.2006.00123.x

[157] Levine, Hagai et al. "Temporal trends in sperm count: a systematic review and meta-regression analysis." Human reproduction update vol. 23,6 (2017): 646-659. doi:10.1093/humupd/dmx022

[158] Swan, Shanna H. and Stacy Colino. Count Down: How Our Modern World Is Threatening Sperm Counts, Altering Male and Female Reproductive Development, and Imperiling the Future of the Human Race. Scribner, 2021.

[159] Huang, Chuan et al. "Decline in semen quality among 30,636 young Chinese men from 2001 to 2015." Fertility and sterility vol. 107,1 (2017): 83-88.e2. doi:10.1016/j.fertnstert.2016.09.035

[160] Cariati, Federica et al. "The evolving role of genetic tests in reproductive medicine." Journal of translational medicine vol. 17,1 267. 14 Aug. 2019, doi:10.1186/s12967-019-2019-8

[161] Koedooder, Rivka et al. "Identification and evaluation of the microbiome in the female and male reproductive tracts." Human reproduction update vol. 25,3 (2019): 298-325. doi:10.1093/humupd/dmy048

[162] Hou, Dongsheng et al. "Microbiota of the seminal fluid from healthy and infertile men." Fertility and sterility vol. 100,5 (2013): 1261-9. doi:10.1016/j.fertnstert.2013.07.1991

[163] Tomaiuolo, Rossella et al. "Microbiota and Human Reproduction: The Case of Male Infertility." High-throughput vol. 9,2 10. 13 Apr. 2020, doi:10.3390/ht9020010

[164] Farahani, Linda et al. "The semen microbiome and its impact on sperm function and male fertility: A systematic review and meta-analysis." Andrology vol. 9,1 (2021): 115-144. doi:10.1111/andr.12886

[165] Monteiro, Catarina et al. "Characterization of microbiota in male infertility cases uncovers differences in seminal hyperviscosity and oligoasthenoteratozoospermia possibly correlated with increased prevalence of infectious bacteria." American journal of reproductive immunology (New York, N.Y. : 1989) vol. 79,6 (2018): e12838. doi:10.1111/aji.12838

[166] Agarwal, Ashok et al. "Role of antioxidants in treatment of male infertility: an overview of the literature." Reproductive biomedicine online vol. 8,6 (2004): 616-27. doi:10.1016/s1472-6483(10)61641-0

[167] Scaruffi, Paola et al. "Oral Antioxidant Treatment of Men Significantly Improves the Reproductive Outcome of IVF Cycles." *Journal of clinical medicine* vol. 10,15 3254. 23 Jul. 2021, doi:10.3390/jcm10153254

[168] Moretti, Elena et al. "The presence of bacteria species in semen and sperm quality." Journal of assisted reproduction and genetics vol. 26,1 (2009): 47-56. doi:10.1007/s10815-008-9283-5

[169] Villegas, J et al. "Bacteria induce expression of apoptosis in human spermatozoa." Apoptosis : an international journal on programmed cell death vol. 10,1 (2005): 105-10. doi:10.1007/s10495-005-6065-8

[170] Schuchardt, Larissa, and Jan Rupp. "Chlamydia trachomatis as the Cause of Infectious Infertility: Acute, Repetitive or Persistent Long-Term Infection?." Current topics in microbiology and immunology vol. 412 (2018): 159-182. doi:10.1007/82_2016_15

[171] Wiesenfeld, Harold C et al. "Bacterial vaginosis is a strong predictor of Neisseria gonorrhoeae and Chlamydia trachomatis infection." Clinical infectious diseases : an official publication of the Infectious Diseases Society of America vol. 36,5 (2003): 663-8. doi:10.1086/367658

[172] Gong, Zheng et al. "Lactobacilli inactivate Chlamydia trachomatis through lactic acid but not H2O2." PloS one vol. 9,9 e107758. 12 Sep. 2014, doi:10.1371/journal.pone.0107758

---

[173] Farahani, Linda et al. "The semen microbiome and its impact on sperm function and male fertility: A systematic review and meta-analysis." Andrology vol. 9,1 (2021): 115-144. doi:10.1111/andr.12886

[174] Altmäe, Signe et al. "The seminal microbiome in health and disease." Nature reviews. Urology vol. 16,12 (2019): 703-721. doi:10.1038/s41585-019-0250-y

[175] Pascual, Liliana et al. "Vaginal colonization and activity of the probiotic bacterium Lactobacillus fermentum L23 in a murine model of vaginal tract infection." Journal of medical microbiology vol. 59,Pt 3 (2010): 360-364. doi:10.1099/jmm.0.012583-0

[176] Bhandari, Praveen, and Vijay Prabha. "Evaluation of profertility effect of probiotic Lactobacillus plantarum 2621 in a murine model." The Indian journal of medical research vol. 142,1 (2015): 79-84. doi:10.4103/0971-5916.162127

[177] Petrova, Mariya I et al. "Lactobacillus iners: Friend or Foe?." Trends in microbiology vol. 25,3 (2017): 182-191. doi:10.1016/j.tim.2016.11.007

[178] Mändar, Reet et al. "Seminal microbiome in men with and without prostatitis." International journal of urology : official journal of the Japanese Urological Association vol. 24,3 (2017): 211-216. doi:10.1111/iju.13286

[179] Tomaiuolo, Rossella et al. "Microbiota and Human Reproduction: The Case of Male Infertility." High-throughput vol. 9,2 10. 13 Apr. 2020, doi:10.3390/ht9020010

[180] Hou, Dongsheng et al. "Microbiota of the seminal fluid from healthy and infertile men." Fertility and sterility vol. 100,5 (2013): 1261-9. doi:10.1016/j.fertnstert.2013.07.1991

[181] Tomaiuolo, Rossella et al. "Microbiota and Human Reproduction: The Case of Male Infertility." High-throughput vol. 9,2 10. 13 Apr. 2020, doi:10.3390/ht9020010

[182] Mändar, Reet et al. "Complementary seminovaginal microbiome in couples." Research in microbiology vol. 166,5 (2015): 440-447. doi:10.1016/j.resmic.2015.03.009

[183] Lannon, Sophia M R et al. "Parallel detection of lactobacillus and bacterial vaginosis-associated bacterial DNA in the chorioamnion and vagina of pregnant women at term." The journal of maternal-fetal & neonatal medicine : the official journal of the European Association of Perinatal Medicine, the

Federation of Asia and Oceania Perinatal Societies, the International Society of Perinatal Obstetricians vol. 32,16 (2019): 2702-2710. doi:10.1080/14767058.2018.1446208

[184] Dardmeh, Fereshteh et al. "Lactobacillus rhamnosus PB01 (DSM 14870) supplementation affects markers of sperm kinematic parameters in a diet-induced obesity mice model." PloS one vol. 12,10 e0185964. 10 Oct. 2017, doi:10.1371/journal.pone.0185964

[185] Chen, X L et al. "Antioxidative activity and protective effect of probiotics against high-fat diet-induced sperm damage in rats." Animal : an international journal of animal bioscience vol. 7,2 (2013): 287-92. doi:10.1017/S1751731112001528

[186] Valcarce, D G et al. "Probiotic administration improves sperm quality in asthenozoospermic human donors." Beneficial microbes vol. 8,2 (2017): 193-206. doi:10.3920/BM2016.0122

[187] Barbonetti, Arcangelo et al. "Effect of vaginal probiotic lactobacilli on in vitro-induced sperm lipid peroxidation and its impact on sperm motility and viability." Fertility and sterility vol. 95,8 (2011): 2485-8. doi:10.1016/j.fertnstert.2011.03.066

[188] Poutahidis, Theofilos et al. "Probiotic microbes sustain youthful serum testosterone levels and testicular size in aging mice." PloS one vol. 9,1 e84877. 2 Jan. 2014, doi:10.1371/journal.pone.0084877

[189] Gibson, Glenn R et al. "Expert consensus document: The International Scientific Association for Probiotics and Prebiotics (ISAPP) consensus statement on the definition and scope of prebiotics." *Nature reviews. Gastroenterology & hepatology* vol. 14,8 (2017): 491-502. doi:10.1038/nrgastro.2017.75

[190] Tomaiuolo, Rossella et al. "Microbiota and Human Reproduction: The Case of Male Infertility." High-throughput vol. 9,2 10. 13 Apr. 2020, doi:10.3390/ht9020010

[191] Maretti, C, and G Cavallini. "The association of a probiotic with a prebiotic (Flortec, Bracco) to improve the quality/quantity of spermatozoa in infertile patients with idiopathic oligoasthenoteratospermia: a pilot study." Andrology vol. 5,3 (2017): 439-444. doi:10.1111/andr.12336

[192] Tomaiuolo, Rossella et al. "Microbiota and Human Reproduction: The Case of Male Infertility." High-throughput vol. 9,2 10. 13 Apr. 2020, doi:10.3390/ht9020010

[193] Hales, Craig M et al. "Prevalence of Obesity and Severe Obesity Among Adults: United States, 2017-2018." NCHS data brief ,360 (2020): 1-8.

[194] Levine, Hagai et al. "Temporal trends in sperm count: a systematic review and meta-regression analysis." Human reproduction update vol. 23,6 (2017): 646-659. doi:10.1093/humupd/dmx022

[195] Palmer, Nicole O et al. "Impact of obesity on male fertility, sperm function and molecular composition." Spermatogenesis vol. 2,4 (2012): 253-263. doi:10.4161/spmg.21362

[196] MacDonald, A A et al. "The impact of body mass index on semen parameters and reproductive hormones in human males: a systematic review with meta-analysis." Human reproduction update vol. 16,3 (2010): 293-311. doi:10.1093/humupd/dmp047

[197] Palmer, Nicole O et al. "Impact of obesity on male fertility, sperm function and molecular composition." Spermatogenesis vol. 2,4 (2012): 253-263. doi:10.4161/spmg.21362

[198] Sermondade, N et al. "BMI in relation to sperm count: an updated systematic review and collaborative meta-analysis." Human reproduction update vol. 19,3 (2013): 221-31. doi:10.1093/humupd/dms050

[199] Bieniek, Jared M et al. "Influence of increasing body mass index on semen and reproductive hormonal parameters in a multi-institutional cohort of subfertile men." Fertility and sterility vol. 106,5 (2016): 1070-1075. doi:10.1016/j.fertnstert.2016.06.041

[200] Kozopas, Nataliia Mykhailivna et al. "Body Mass Index and Sperm Quality: Is there a Relationship?." Journal of human reproductive sciences vol. 13,2 (2020): 110-113. doi:10.4103/jhrs.JHRS_15_20

[201] Palmer, Nicole O et al. "Impact of obesity on male fertility, sperm function and molecular composition." Spermatogenesis vol. 2,4 (2012): 253-263. doi:10.4161/spmg.21362

[202] Fui, Mark Ng Tang et al. "Lowered testosterone in male obesity: mechanisms, morbidity and management." Asian journal of andrology vol. 16,2 (2014): 223-31. doi:10.4103/1008-682X.122365

---

[203] Mir, J et al. "Impact of weight loss on sperm DNA integrity in obese men." Andrologia, 10.1111/and.12957. 1 Feb. 2018, doi:10.1111/and.12957

[204] Yang, Qingling et al. "Effect of paternal overweight or obesity on IVF treatment outcomes and the possible mechanisms involved." Scientific reports vol. 6 29787. 14 Jul. 2016, doi:10.1038/srep29787

[205] Desai, Nisarg et al. "Free radical theory of aging: implications in male infertility." Urology vol. 75,1 (2010): 14-9. doi:10.1016/j.urology.2009.05.025

[206] Cai, Hui et al. "Responses and coping methods of different testicular cell types to heat stress: overview and perspectives." Bioscience reports vol. 41,6 (2021): BSR20210443. doi:10.1042/BSR20210443

[207] Tremellen, Kelton et al. "Metabolic endotoxaemia related inflammation is associated with hypogonadism in overweight men." Basic and clinical andrology vol. 27 5. 8 Mar. 2017, doi:10.1186/s12610-017-0049-8

[208] Jurewicz, Joanna et al. "Dietary Patterns and Their Relationship With Semen Quality." American journal of men's health vol. 12,3 (2018): 575-583. doi:10.1177/1557988315627139

[209] Merhi, Zaher O et al. "Male adiposity impairs clinical pregnancy rate by in vitro fertilization without affecting day 3 embryo quality." Obesity (Silver Spring, Md.) vol. 21,8 (2013): 1608-12. doi:10.1002/oby.20164

[210] Palmer, Nicole O et al. "Impact of obesity on male fertility, sperm function and molecular composition." Spermatogenesis vol. 2,4 (2012): 253-263. doi:10.4161/spmg.21362

[211] Nguyen, Ruby H N et al. "Men's body mass index and infertility." Human reproduction (Oxford, England) vol. 22,9 (2007): 2488-93. doi:10.1093/humrep/dem139

[212] Håkonsen, Linn Berger et al. "Does weight loss improve semen quality and reproductive hormones? Results from a cohort of severely obese men." Reproductive health vol. 8 24. 17 Aug. 2011, doi:10.1186/1742-4755-8-24

[213] Mir, J et al. "Impact of weight loss on sperm DNA integrity in obese men." Andrologia, 10.1111/and.12957. 1 Feb. 2018, doi:10.1111/and.12957

[214] Palmer, Nicole O et al. "Diet and exercise in an obese mouse fed a high-fat diet improve metabolic health and reverse perturbed sperm function." American journal of physiology. Endocrinology and metabolism vol. 302,7 (2012): E768-80. doi:10.1152/ajpendo.00401.2011

[215] Pearce, Karma L, and Kelton Tremellen. "The Effect of Macronutrients on Reproductive Hormones in Overweight and Obese Men: A Pilot Study." Nutrients vol. 11,12 3059. 14 Dec. 2019, doi:10.3390/nu11123059

[216] Salas-Huetos, Albert et al. "Male adiposity, sperm parameters and reproductive hormones: An updated systematic review and collaborative meta-analysis." Obesity reviews : an official journal of the International Association for the Study of Obesity vol. 22,1 (2021): e13082. doi:10.1111/obr.13082

[217] Nordkap, Loa et al. "Psychological stress and testicular function: a cross-sectional study of 1,215 Danish men." Fertility and sterility vol. 105,1 (2016): 174-87.e1-2. doi:10.1016/j.fertnstert.2015.09.016

[218] Radwan, M et al. "Sperm DNA damage-the effect of stress and everyday life factors." International journal of impotence research vol. 28,4 (2016): 148-54. doi:10.1038/ijir.2016.15

[219] Qu, Fan et al. "The association between psychological stress and miscarriage: A systematic review and meta-analysis." Scientific reports vol. 7,1 1731. 11 May. 2017, doi:10.1038/s41598-017-01792-3

[220] Domar, A D et al. "Impact of group psychological interventions on pregnancy rates in infertile women." Fertility and sterility vol. 73,4 (2000): 805-11. doi:10.1016/s0015-0282(99)00493-8

[221] Sharma, Rakesh et al. "Lifestyle factors and reproductive health: taking control of your fertility." Reproductive biology and endocrinology : RB&E vol. 11 66. 16 Jul. 2013, doi:10.1186/1477-7827-11-66

[222] Holmboe, Stine Agergaard et al. "Use of e-cigarettes associated with lower sperm counts in a cross-sectional study of young men from the general population." Human reproduction (Oxford, England) vol. 35,7 (2020): 1693-1701. doi:10.1093/humrep/deaa089

[223] Biviá-Roig, Gemma et al. "Impact of the COVID-19 Pandemic on the Lifestyles and Quality of Life of Women With Fertility Problems: A Cross-Sectional Study." Frontiers in public health vol. 9 686115. 19 Jul. 2021, doi:10.3389/fpubh.2021.686115

[224] Carroll, K et al. "Marijuana use and its influence on sperm morphology and motility: identified risk for fertility among Jamaican men." Andrology vol. 8,1 (2020): 136-142. doi:10.1111/andr.12670

[225] Mueller, B A et al. "Recreational drug use and the risk of primary infertility." Epidemiology (Cambridge, Mass.) vol. 1,3 (1990): 195-200. doi:10.1097/00001648-199005000-00003

[226] Marić, Tihana et al. "Environmental and occupational exposures associated with male infertility." Arhiv za higijenu rada i toksikologiju vol. 72,3 101-113. 28 Jun. 2021, doi:10.2478/aiht-2021-72-3510

[227] Maya-Enero, Silvia et al. "Neurocognitive and behavioral profile of fetal alcohol spectrum disorder." Anales de pediatria vol. 95,3 (2021): 208.e1-208.e9. doi:10.1016/j.anpede.2020.12.012

[228] Ding, Jiayi et al. "FDA-approved medications that impair human spermatogenesis." Oncotarget vol. 8,6 (2017): 10714-10725. doi:10.18632/oncotarget.12956

[229] Casilla-Lennon, Marianne M et al. "The effect of antidepressants on fertility." American journal of obstetrics and gynecology vol. 215,3 (2016): 314.e1-5. doi:10.1016/j.ajog.2016.01.170

[230] Drobnis, Erma Z, and Ajay K Nangia. "Pain Medications and Male Reproduction." Advances in experimental medicine and biology vol. 1034 (2017): 39-57. doi:10.1007/978-3-319-69535-8_6

[231] Sharma, Rakesh et al. "Lifestyle factors and reproductive health: taking control of your fertility." Reproductive biology and endocrinology : RB&E vol. 11 66. 16 Jul. 2013, doi:10.1186/1477-7827-11-66

[232] Bieniek, Jared M, and Kirk C Lo. "Recent advances in understanding & managing male infertility." F1000Research vol. 5 2756. 24 Nov. 2016, doi:10.12688/f1000research.9375.1

[233] Cariati, Federica et al. ""Bisphenol a: an emerging threat to male fertility"." Reproductive biology and endocrinology : RB&E vol. 17,1 6. 20 Jan. 2019, doi:10.1186/s12958-018-0447-6

[234] Matthews, T J, and Brady E Hamilton. "Delayed childbearing: more women are having their first child later in life." *NCHS data brief*,21 (2009): 1-8.

[235] Braga, Daniela Paes Almeida Ferreira et al. "The impact of food intake and social habits on embryo quality and the likelihood of blastocyst formation." Reproductive biomedicine online vol. 31,1 (2015): 30-8. doi:10.1016/j.rbmo.2015.03.007

---

[236] Maldonado-Cárceles, Ana B et al. "Dietary patterns and ovarian reserve among women attending a fertility clinic." Fertility and sterility vol. 114,3 (2020): 610-617. doi:10.1016/j.fertnstert.2020.04.030

[237] Fontana, Roberta, and Sara Della Torre. "The Deep Correlation between Energy Metabolism and Reproduction: A View on the Effects of Nutrition for Women Fertility." *Nutrients* vol. 8,2 87. 11 Feb. 2016, doi:10.3390/nu8020087

[238] Garruti, Gabriella et al. "Weighing the Impact of Diet and Lifestyle on Female Reproductive Function." Current medicinal chemistry vol. 26,19 (2019): 3584-3592. doi:10.2174/0929867324666170518101008

[239] Karayiannis, Dimitrios et al. "Adherence to the Mediterranean diet and IVF success rate among non-obese women attempting fertility." Human reproduction (Oxford, England) vol. 33,3 (2018): 494-502. doi:10.1093/humrep/dey003

[240] Fontana, Roberta, and Sara Della Torre. "The Deep Correlation between Energy Metabolism and Reproduction: A View on the Effects of Nutrition for Women Fertility." *Nutrients* vol. 8,2 87. 11 Feb. 2016, doi:10.3390/nu8020087

[241] Cirillo, Michela et al. "The effects of COVID-19 lockdown on lifestyle and emotional state in women undergoing assisted reproductive technology: Results of an Italian survey." Journal of gynecology obstetrics and human reproduction vol. 50,8 (2021): 102079. doi:10.1016/j.jogoh.2021.102079

[242] Gaskins, Audrey J et al. "Dietary patterns and outcomes of assisted reproduction." *American journal of obstetrics and gynecology* vol. 220,6 (2019): 567.e1-567.e18. doi:10.1016/j.ajog.2019.02.004

[243] Eskew, Ashley M et al. "Dietary patterns are associated with improved ovarian reserve in overweight and obese women: a cross-sectional study of the Lifestyle and Ovarian Reserve (LORe) cohort." *Reproductive biology and endocrinology : RB&E* vol. 20,1 33. 19 Feb. 2022, doi:10.1186/s12958-022-00907-4

[244] https://www.hsph.harvard.edu/nutritionsource/nurses-health-study/

[245] https://ajph.aphapublications.org/toc/ajph/106/9

[246] Chavarro, Jorge E et al. "Diet and lifestyle in the prevention of ovulatory disorder infertility." Obstetrics and gynecology vol. 110,5 (2007): 1050-8. doi:10.1097/01.AOG.0000287293.25465.e1

---

[247] Karayiannis, Dimitrios et al. "Association between adherence to the Mediterranean diet and semen quality parameters in male partners of couples attempting fertility." Human reproduction (Oxford, England) vol. 32,1 (2017): 215-222. doi:10.1093/humrep/dew288

[248] Jurewicz, Joanna et al. "Dietary Patterns and Their Relationship With Semen Quality." American journal of men's health vol. 12,3 (2018): 575-583. doi:10.1177/1557988315627139

[249] Gaskins, Audrey J et al. "Dietary patterns and semen quality in young men." Human reproduction (Oxford, England) vol. 27,10 (2012): 2899-907. doi:10.1093/humrep/des298

[250] Cutillas-Tolín, A et al. "Mediterranean and western dietary patterns are related to markers of testicular function among healthy men." Human reproduction (Oxford, England) vol. 30,12 (2015): 2945-55. doi:10.1093/humrep/dev236

[251] Salas-Huetos, Albert et al. "Dietary patterns, foods and nutrients in male fertility parameters and fecundability: a systematic review of observational studies." Human reproduction update vol. 23,4 (2017): 371-389. doi:10.1093/humupd/dmx006

[252] Efrat, Michal et al. "Dietary patterns are positively associated with semen quality." Fertility and sterility vol. 109,5 (2018): 809-816. doi:10.1016/j.fertnstert.2018.01.010

[253] Vujkovic, Marijana et al. "The preconception Mediterranean dietary pattern in couples undergoing in vitro fertilization/intracytoplasmic sperm injection treatment increases the chance of pregnancy." Fertility and sterility vol. 94,6 (2010): 2096-101. doi:10.1016/j.fertnstert.2009.12.079

[254] Pearce, Karma L, and Kelton Tremellen. "The Effect of Macronutrients on Reproductive Hormones in Overweight and Obese Men: A Pilot Study." Nutrients vol. 11,12 3059. 14 Dec. 2019, doi:10.3390/nu11123059

[255] Wu, Guoyao. "Dietary protein intake and human health." *Food & function* vol. 7,3 (2016): 1251-65. doi:10.1039/c5fo01530h

[256] Elango, Rajavel, and Ronald O Ball. "Protein and Amino Acid Requirements during Pregnancy." *Advances in nutrition (Bethesda, Md.)* vol. 7,4 839S-44S. 15 Jul. 2016, doi:10.3945/an.115.011817

[257] Sun, Yangbo et al. "Association of Major Dietary Protein Sources With All-Cause and Cause-Specific Mortality: Prospective Cohort Study." *Journal*

of the American Heart Association vol. 10,5 (2021): e015553. doi:10.1161/JAHA.119.015553

[258] Guzmán, Carolina et al. "Maternal protein restriction during pregnancy and/or lactation negatively affects follicular ovarian development and steroidogenesis in the prepubertal rat offspring." Archives of medical research vol. 45,4 (2014): 294-300. doi:10.1016/j.arcmed.2014.05.005

[259] Souter, I et al. "The association of protein intake (amount and type) with ovarian antral follicle counts among infertile women: results from the EARTH prospective study cohort." BJOG : an international journal of obstetrics and gynaecology vol. 124,10 (2017): 1547-1555. doi:10.1111/1471-0528.14630

[260] Chavarro, Jorge E et al. "Protein intake and ovulatory infertility." *American journal of obstetrics and gynecology* vol. 198,2 (2008): 210.e1-7. doi:10.1016/j.ajog.2007.06.057

[261] Mumford, S. L., A. Alohali, and J. Wactawski-Wende. "Dietary protein intake and reproductive hormones and ovulation: the BioCycle study." *Fertility and Sterility* 104.3 (2015): e2.

[262] Vanegas, Jose C et al. "Soy food intake and treatment outcomes of women undergoing assisted reproductive technology." *Fertility and sterility* vol. 103,3 (2015): 749-55.e2. doi:10.1016/j.fertnstert.2014.12.104

[263] Unfer, Vittorio et al. "Phytoestrogens may improve the pregnancy rate in in vitro fertilization-embryo transfer cycles: a prospective, controlled, randomized trial." *Fertility and sterility* vol. 82,6 (2004): 1509-13. doi:10.1016/j.fertnstert.2004.07.934

[264] Pearce, Karma L, and Kelton Tremellen. "The Effect of Macronutrients on Reproductive Hormones in Overweight and Obese Men: A Pilot Study." Nutrients vol. 11,12 3059. 14 Dec. 2019, doi:10.3390/nu11123059

[265] Chavarro, Jorge E et al. "Soy food and isoflavone intake in relation to semen quality parameters among men from an infertility clinic." Human reproduction (Oxford, England) vol. 23,11 (2008): 2584-90. doi:10.1093/humrep/den243

[266] https://www.health.harvard.edu/diseases-and-conditions/the-lowdown-on-glycemic-index-and-glycemic-load

[267] Silvestris, Erica et al. "Nutrition and Female Fertility: An Interdependent Correlation." Frontiers in endocrinology vol. 10 346. 7 Jun. 2019, doi:10.3389/fendo.2019.00346

[268] Chavarro, J E et al. "A prospective study of dietary carbohydrate quantity and quality in relation to risk of ovulatory infertility." European journal of clinical nutrition vol. 63,1 (2009): 78-86. doi:10.1038/sj.ejcn.1602904

[269] Willis, Sydney K et al. "Glycemic load, dietary fiber, and added sugar and fecundability in 2 preconception cohorts." The American journal of clinical nutrition vol. 112,1 (2020): 27-38. doi:10.1093/ajcn/nqz312

[270] Gaskins, Audrey J et al. "Maternal whole grain intake and outcomes of in vitro fertilization." Fertility and sterility vol. 105,6 (2016): 1503-1510.e4. doi:10.1016/j.fertnstert.2016.02.015

[271] Machtinger, Ronit et al. "Association between preconception maternal beverage intake and in vitro fertilization outcomes." Fertility and sterility vol. 108,6 (2017): 1026-1033. doi:10.1016/j.fertnstert.2017.09.007

[272] Setti, Amanda Souza et al. "Is there an association between artificial sweetener consumption and assisted reproduction outcomes?." Reproductive biomedicine online vol. 36,2 (2018): 145-153. doi:10.1016/j.rbmo.2017.11.004

[273] Ricci, E et al. "Dietary habits and semen parameters: a systematic narrative review." Andrology vol. 6,1 (2018): 104-116. doi:10.1111/andr.12452

[274] Chiu, Y H et al. "Sugar-sweetened beverage intake in relation to semen quality and reproductive hormone levels in young men." Human reproduction (Oxford, England) vol. 29,7 (2014): 1575-84. doi:10.1093/humrep/deu102

[275] Pearce, Karma L, and Kelton Tremellen. "The Effect of Macronutrients on Reproductive Hormones in Overweight and Obese Men: A Pilot Study." Nutrients vol. 11,12 3059. 14 Dec. 2019, doi:10.3390/nu11123059

[276] Caronia, Lisa M et al. "Abrupt decrease in serum testosterone levels after an oral glucose load in men: implications for screening for hypogonadism." Clinical endocrinology vol. 78,2 (2013): 291-6. doi:10.1111/j.1365-2265.2012.04486.x

[277] Ricci, E et al. "Dietary habits and semen parameters: a systematic narrative review." Andrology vol. 6,1 (2018): 104-116. doi:10.1111/andr.12452

[278] Madej, Dawid et al. "Influence of Fruit and Vegetable Consumption on Antioxidant Status and Semen Quality: A Cross-Sectional Study in Adult Men." *Frontiers in nutrition* vol. 8 753843. 15 Oct. 2021, doi:10.3389/fnut.2021.753843

[279] Hohos, Natalie M, and Malgorzata E Skaznik-Wikiel. "High-Fat Diet and Female Fertility." Endocrinology vol. 158,8 (2017): 2407-2419. doi:10.1210/en.2017-00371

[280] Jensen, Tina K et al. "High dietary intake of saturated fat is associated with reduced semen quality among 701 young Danish men from the general population." The American journal of clinical nutrition vol. 97,2 (2013): 411-8. doi:10.3945/ajcn.112.042432

[281] Attaman, Jill A et al. "Dietary fat and semen quality among men attending a fertility clinic." Human reproduction (Oxford, England) vol. 27,5 (2012): 1466-74. doi:10.1093/humrep/des065

[282] Skoracka, Kinga et al. "Female Fertility and the Nutritional Approach: The Most Essential Aspects." *Advances in nutrition (Bethesda, Md.)* vol. 12,6 (2021): 2372-2386. doi:10.1093/advances/nmab068

[283] Chavarro, Jorge E et al. "Trans-fatty acid levels in sperm are associated with sperm concentration among men from an infertility clinic." Fertility and sterility vol. 95,5 (2011): 1794-7. doi:10.1016/j.fertnstert.2010.10.039

[284] Skoracka, Kinga et al. "Female Fertility and the Nutritional Approach: The Most Essential Aspects." Advances in nutrition (Bethesda, Md.) vol. 12,6 (2021): 2372-2386. doi:10.1093/advances/nmab068

[285] Simopoulos, A P. "The importance of the ratio of omega-6/omega-3 essential fatty acids." *Biomedicine & pharmacotherapy = Biomedecine & pharmacotherapie* vol. 56,8 (2002): 365-79. doi:10.1016/s0753-3322(02)00253-6

[286] Stanhiser, Jamie et al. "Serum omega-3 and omega-6 fatty acid concentrations and natural fertility." Human reproduction (Oxford, England) vol. 35,4 (2020): 950-957. doi:10.1093/humrep/dez305

[287] Jungheim, Emily S et al. "Relationship between serum polyunsaturated fatty acids and pregnancy in women undergoing in vitro fertilization." The Journal of clinical endocrinology and metabolism vol. 98,8 (2013): E1364-8. doi:10.1210/jc.2012-4115

[288] Stanhiser, Jamie et al. "Serum omega-3 and omega-6 fatty acid concentrations and natural fertility." *Human reproduction (Oxford, England)* vol. 35,4 (2020): 950-957. doi:10.1093/humrep/dez305

[289] Al-Safi, Zain A et al. "Omega-3 Fatty Acid Supplementation Lowers Serum FSH in Normal Weight But Not Obese Women." *The Journal of clinical endocrinology and metabolism* vol. 101,1 (2016): 324-33. doi:10.1210/jc.2015-2913

[290] Koga, Fumitoshi et al. "Relationship between nutrition and reproduction." Reproductive medicine and biology vol. 19,3 254-264. 15 Jun. 2020, doi:10.1002/rmb2.12332

[291] Chiu, Y-H et al. "Serum omega-3 fatty acids and treatment outcomes among women undergoing assisted reproduction." Human reproduction (Oxford, England) vol. 33,1 (2018): 156-165. doi:10.1093/humrep/dex335

[292] Collodel, Giulia et al. "Relevance of Fatty Acids to Sperm Maturation and Quality." Oxidative medicine and cellular longevity vol. 2020 7038124. 5 Feb. 2020, doi:10.1155/2020/7038124

[293] Jensen, Tina Kold et al. "Associations of Fish Oil Supplement Use With Testicular Function in Young Men." JAMA network open vol. 3,1 e1919462. 3 Jan. 2020, doi:10.1001/jamanetworkopen.2019.19462

[294] MInguez-Alarcón, Lidia et al. "Fatty acid intake in relation to reproductive hormones and testicular volume among young healthy men." Asian journal of andrology vol. 19,2 (2017): 184-190. doi:10.4103/1008-682X.190323

[295] Agostoni, Carlo et al. "Whole blood fatty acid composition at birth: from the maternal compartment to the infant." *Clinical nutrition (Edinburgh, Scotland)* vol. 30,4 (2011): 503-5. doi:10.1016/j.clnu.2011.01.016

[296] Cánovas-Conesa, A et al. The association of adherence to a Mediterranean diet during early pregnancy and the risk of gastroschisis in the offspring. *Cirugia pediatrica : organo oficial de la Sociedad Espanola de Cirugia Pediatrica* vol. 26,1 (2013): 37-43.

[297] Chavarro, Jorge E et al. "Dietary fatty acid intakes and the risk of ovulatory infertility." *The American journal of clinical nutrition* vol. 85,1 (2007): 231-7. doi:10.1093/ajcn/85.1.231

[298] Chavarro, J.E. et al. "Dietary fat intake and in-vitro fertilization outcomes: saturated fat intake is associated with fewer metaphase 2 oocytes."

Human Reproduction, Volume 27, Issue suppl_2, 2012, Pages ii78–ii79, https://doi.org/10.1093/humrep/27.s2.52

[299] Mumford, Sunni L et al. "Preconception Plasma Phospholipid Fatty Acids and Fecundability." *The Journal of clinical endocrinology and metabolism* vol. 103,12 (2018): 4501-4510. doi:10.1210/jc.2018-00448

[300] Sińska, Beata et al. "Znaczenie diety w optymalizacji płodności kobiety" [The diet in improving fertility in women]. *Polski merkuriusz lekarski : organ Polskiego Towarzystwa Lekarskiego* vol. 36,216 (2014): 400-2.

[301] https://onlinelibrary.wiley.com/doi/full/10.1111/andr.12452#andr12452-tbl-0005

[302] Ricci, E et al. "Dietary habits and semen parameters: a systematic narrative review." Andrology vol. 6,1 (2018): 104-116. doi:10.1111/andr.12452

[303] Eslamian, Ghazaleh et al. "Intake of food groups and idiopathic asthenozoospermia: a case-control study." Human reproduction (Oxford, England) vol. 27,11 (2012): 3328-36. doi:10.1093/humrep/des311

[304] Xia, Wei et al. "Men's meat intake and treatment outcomes among couples undergoing assisted reproduction." Fertility and sterility vol. 104,4 (2015): 972-979. doi:10.1016/j.fertnstert.2015.06.037

[305] Ricci, E et al. "Dietary habits and semen parameters: a systematic narrative review." Andrology vol. 6,1 (2018): 104-116. doi:10.1111/andr.12452

[306] Gaskins, Audrey J et al. "Seafood Intake, Sexual Activity, and Time to Pregnancy." *The Journal of clinical endocrinology and metabolism* vol. 103,7 (2018): 2680-2688. doi:10.1210/jc.2018-00385

[307] Hsi, Hsing-Cheng et al. "Methylmercury Concentration in Fish and Risk-Benefit Assessment of Fish Intake among Pregnant versus Infertile Women in Taiwan." *PloS one* vol. 11,5 e0155704. 17 May. 2016, doi:10.1371/journal.pone.0155704

[308] https://www.thoughtco.com/dairy-farming-ancient-history-171199

[309] Afeiche, M et al. "Dairy food intake in relation to semen quality and reproductive hormone levels among physically active young men." Human reproduction (Oxford, England) vol. 28,8 (2013): 2265-75. doi:10.1093/humrep/det133

[310] Afeiche, Myriam C et al. "Dairy intake and semen quality among men attending a fertility clinic." Fertility and sterility vol. 101,5 (2014): 1280-7. doi:10.1016/j.fertnstert.2014.02.003

[311] Eslamian, Ghazaleh et al. "Intake of food groups and idiopathic asthenozoospermia: a case-control study." Human reproduction (Oxford, England) vol. 27,11 (2012): 3328-36. doi:10.1093/humrep/des311

[312] Ricci, E et al. "Dietary habits and semen parameters: a systematic narrative review." Andrology vol. 6,1 (2018): 104-116. doi:10.1111/andr.12452

[313] Pearce, Karma L, and Kelton Tremellen. "The Effect of Macronutrients on Reproductive Hormones in Overweight and Obese Men: A Pilot Study." Nutrients vol. 11,12 3059. 14 Dec. 2019, doi:10.3390/nu11123059

[314] Chavarro, J E et al. "A prospective study of dairy foods intake and anovulatory infertility." *Human reproduction (Oxford, England)* vol. 22,5 (2007): 1340-7. doi:10.1093/humrep/dem019

[315] Wise, Lauren A et al. "Dairy intake and fecundability in 2 preconception cohort studies." *The American journal of clinical nutrition* vol. 105,1 (2017): 100-110. doi:10.3945/ajcn.116.138404

[316] https://ods.od.nih.gov/HealthInformation/Dietary_Reference_Intakes.aspx

[317] https://www.nccih.nih.gov/health/vitamins-and-minerals

[318] https://www.dietaryguidelines.gov/

[319] https://www.dietaryguidelines.gov/

[320] https://www.myplate.gov/

[321] Ramakrishnan, Usha et al. "Effect of women's nutrition before and during early pregnancy on maternal and infant outcomes: a systematic review." Paediatric and perinatal epidemiology vol. 26 Suppl 1 (2012): 285-301. doi:10.1111/j.1365-3016.2012.01281.x

[322] Mousa, Aya et al. "Macronutrient and Micronutrient Intake during Pregnancy: An Overview of Recent Evidence." Nutrients vol. 11,2 443. 20 Feb. 2019, doi:10.3390/nu11020443

[323] Mousa, Aya et al. "Macronutrient and Micronutrient Intake during Pregnancy: An Overview of Recent Evidence." Nutrients vol. 11,2 443. 20 Feb. 2019, doi:10.3390/nu11020443

---

[324] Adams, James B et al. "Evidence-Based Recommendations for an Optimal Prenatal Supplement for Women in the U.S., Part Two: Minerals." Nutrients vol. 13,6 1849. 28 May. 2021, doi:10.3390/nu13061849

[325] Santander Ballestín, Sonia et al. "Is Supplementation with Micronutrients Still Necessary during Pregnancy? A Review." Nutrients vol. 13,9 3134. 8 Sep. 2021, doi:10.3390/nu13093134

[326] Adams, James B et al. "Evidence-Based Recommendations for an Optimal Prenatal Supplement for Women in the U.S., Part Two: Minerals." Nutrients vol. 13,6 1849. 28 May. 2021, doi:10.3390/nu13061849

[327] Adams, James B et al. "Evidence-Based Recommendations for an Optimal Prenatal Supplement for Women in the U.S., Part Two: Minerals." Nutrients vol. 13,6 1849. 28 May. 2021, doi:10.3390/nu13061849

[328] Adams, James B et al. "Evidence-Based Recommendations for an Optimal Prenatal Supplement for Women in the U.S., Part Two: Minerals." Nutrients vol. 13,6 1849. 28 May. 2021, doi:10.3390/nu13061849

[329] Adams, James B et al. "Evidence-Based Recommendations for an Optimal Prenatal Supplement for Women in the U.S., Part Two: Minerals." Nutrients vol. 13,6 1849. 28 May. 2021, doi:10.3390/nu13061849

[330] Cetin, I et al. "Role of micronutrients in the periconceptional period." Human reproduction update vol. 16,1 (2010): 80-95. doi:10.1093/humupd/dmp025

[331] Schaefer, Ella, and Deborah Nock. "The Impact of Preconceptional Multiple-Micronutrient Supplementation on Female Fertility." Clinical medicine insights. Women's health vol. 12 1179562X19843868. 23 Apr. 2019, doi:10.1177/1179562X19843868

[332] Ruder, Elizabeth H et al. "Impact of oxidative stress on female fertility." Current opinion in obstetrics & gynecology vol. 21,3 (2009): 219-22. doi:10.1097/gco.0b013e32832924ba

[333] Agarwal, Ashok et al. "The effects of oxidative stress on female reproduction: a review." Reproductive biology and endocrinology : RB&E vol. 10 49. 29 Jun. 2012, doi:10.1186/1477-7827-10-49

[334] Ebisch, I M W et al. "The importance of folate, zinc and antioxidants in the pathogenesis and prevention of subfertility." Human reproduction update vol. 13,2 (2007): 163-74. doi:10.1093/humupd/dml054

[335] Ruder, Elizabeth H et al. "Oxidative stress and antioxidants: exposure and impact on female fertility." Human reproduction update vol. 14,4 (2008): 345-57. doi:10.1093/humupd/dmn011

[336] Agarwal, Ashok et al. "Utility of Antioxidants in the Treatment of Male Infertility: Clinical Guidelines Based on a Systematic Review and Analysis of Evidence." The world journal of men's health vol. 39,2 (2021): 233-290. doi:10.5534/wjmh.200196

[337] Mozaffarian, Dariush. "Dietary and Policy Priorities for Cardiovascular Disease, Diabetes, and Obesity: A Comprehensive Review." Circulation vol. 133,2 (2016): 187-225. doi:10.1161/CIRCULATIONAHA.115.018585

[338] Pérez-Torres, Israel et al. "Oxidative Stress, Plant Natural Antioxidants, and Obesity." International journal of molecular sciences vol. 22,4 1786. 11 Feb. 2021, doi:10.3390/ijms22041786

[339] Nouri, Kazem et al. "The Impact of a Standardized Oral Multinutrient Supplementation on Embryo Quality in in vitro Fertilization/Intracytoplasmic Sperm Injection: A Prospective Randomized Trial." Gynecologic and obstetric investigation vol. 82,1 (2017): 8-14. doi:10.1159/000452662

[340] Luddi, Alice et al. "Antioxidants reduce oxidative stress in follicular fluid of aged women undergoing IVF." Reproductive biology and endocrinology : RB&E vol. 14,1 57. 7 Sep. 2016, doi:10.1186/s12958-016-0184-7

[341] Ruder, Elizabeth H et al. "Female dietary antioxidant intake and time to pregnancy among couples treated for unexplained infertility." Fertility and sterility vol. 101,3 (2014): 759-66. doi:10.1016/j.fertnstert.2013.11.008

[342] Westphal, Lynn M et al. "A nutritional supplement for improving fertility in women: a pilot study." The Journal of reproductive medicine vol. 49,4 (2004): 289-93.

[343] Westphal, L M et al. "Double-blind, placebo-controlled study of Fertilityblend: a nutritional supplement for improving fertility in women." Clinical and experimental obstetrics & gynecology vol. 33,4 (2006): 205-8.

[344] Showell, Marian G et al. "Antioxidants for female subfertility." The Cochrane database of systematic reviews vol. 8,8 CD007807. 27 Aug. 2020, doi:10.1002/14651858.CD007807.pub4

[345] Agrawal, Rina et al. "Prospective randomized trial of multiple micronutrients in subfertile women undergoing ovulation induction: a pilot

study." Reproductive biomedicine online vol. 24,1 (2012): 54-60. doi:10.1016/j.rbmo.2011.10.004

[346] Agarwal, Ashok et al. "Utility of Antioxidants in the Treatment of Male Infertility: Clinical Guidelines Based on a Systematic Review and Analysis of Evidence." The world journal of men's health vol. 39,2 (2021): 233-290. doi:10.5534/wjmh.200196

[347] Agarwal, Ashok et al. "Role of antioxidants in treatment of male infertility: an overview of the literature." Reproductive biomedicine online vol. 8,6 (2004): 616-27. doi:10.1016/s1472-6483(10)61641-0

[348] Carlsen, E et al. "Evidence for decreasing quality of semen during past 50 years." BMJ (Clinical research ed.) vol. 305,6854 (1992): 609-13. doi:10.1136/bmj.305.6854.609

[349] Rahimlou, Mehran et al. "Dietary Antioxidant Intake in Relation to Semen Quality Parameters in Infertile Men: a Cross-Sectional Study." Clinical nutrition research vol. 8,3 229-237. 25 Jul. 2019, doi:10.7762/cnr.2019.8.3.229

[350] Palmer, Nicole O et al. "Impact of obesity on male fertility, sperm function and molecular composition." Spermatogenesis vol. 2,4 (2012): 253-263. doi:10.4161/spmg.21362

[351] Scaruffi, Paola et al. "Oral Antioxidant Treatment of Men Significantly Improves the Reproductive Outcome of IVF Cycles." *Journal of clinical medicine* vol. 10,15 3254. 23 Jul. 2021, doi:10.3390/jcm10153254

[352] Agarwal, Ashok et al. "Role of antioxidants in treatment of male infertility: an overview of the literature." Reproductive biomedicine online vol. 8,6 (2004): 616-27. doi:10.1016/s1472-6483(10)61641-0

[353] Rahimlou, Mehran et al. "Dietary Antioxidant Intake in Relation to Semen Quality Parameters in Infertile Men: a Cross-Sectional Study." Clinical nutrition research vol. 8,3 229-237. 25 Jul. 2019, doi:10.7762/cnr.2019.8.3.229

[354] https://ods.od.nih.gov/factsheets/list-all/

[355] Yu, Shuai et al. "β-carotene improves oocyte development and maturation under oxidative stress in vitro." *In vitro cellular & developmental biology. Animal* vol. 55,7 (2019): 548-558. doi:10.1007/s11626-019-00373-0

[356] Rahimlou, Mehran et al. "Dietary Antioxidant Intake in Relation to Semen Quality Parameters in Infertile Men: a Cross-Sectional Study." Clinical nutrition research vol. 8,3 229-237. 25 Jul. 2019, doi:10.7762/cnr.2019.8.3.229

[357] Nouri, Mehran et al. "The effects of lycopene supplement on the spermatogram and seminal oxidative stress in infertile men: A randomized, double-blind, placebo-controlled clinical trial." Phytotherapy research : PTR vol. 33,12 (2019): 3203-3211. doi:10.1002/ptr.6493

[358] Mínguez-Alarcón, Lidia et al. "Dietary intake of antioxidant nutrients is associated with semen quality in young university students." Human reproduction (Oxford, England) vol. 27,9 (2012): 2807-14. doi:10.1093/humrep/des247

[359] https://ods.od.nih.gov/factsheets/VitaminA-Consumer/

[360] Klemmensen, Ak et al. "Intake of vitamin C and E in pregnancy and risk of pre-eclampsia: prospective study among 57 346 women." *BJOG : an international journal of obstetrics and gynaecology* vol. 116,7 (2009): 964-74. doi:10.1111/j.1471-0528.2009.02150.x

[361] Angulo, Constanza et al. "Vitamin C and oxidative stress in the seminiferous epithelium." Biological research vol. 44,2 (2011): 169-80.

[362] Greco, Ermanno et al. "Reduction of the incidence of sperm DNA fragmentation by oral antioxidant treatment." Journal of andrology vol. 26,3 (2005): 349-53. doi:10.2164/jandrol.04146

[363] Rafiee, Bahare et al. "Comparing the Effectiveness of Dietary Vitamin C and Exercise Interventions on Fertility Parameters in Normal Obese Men." Urology journal vol. 13,2 2635-9. 16 Apr. 2016

[364] Li, Ming-Chieh et al. "Men's Intake of Vitamin C and β-Carotene Is Positively Related to Fertilization Rate but Not to Live Birth Rate in Couples Undergoing Infertility Treatment." The Journal of nutrition vol. 149,11 (2019): 1977-1984. doi:10.1093/jn/nxz149

[365] https://ods.od.nih.gov/factsheets/VitaminC-HealthProfessional/

[366] Holick, Michael F, and Tai C Chen. "Vitamin D deficiency: a worldwide problem with health consequences." *The American journal of clinical nutrition* vol. 87,4 (2008): 1080S-6S. doi:10.1093/ajcn/87.4.1080S

[367] Webb, Ann R et al. "Colour Counts: Sunlight and Skin Type as Drivers of Vitamin D Deficiency at UK Latitudes." Nutrients vol. 10,4 457. 7 Apr. 2018, doi:10.3390/nu10040457

---

[368] Lerchbaum, Elisabeth, and Barbara Obermayer-Pietsch. "Vitamin D and fertility: a systematic review." European journal of endocrinology vol. 166,5 (2012): 765-78. doi:10.1530/EJE-11-0984

[369] Atanasovska, Emilija et al. "Vitamin D levels and oxidative stress markers in patients hospitalized with COVID-19." *Redox report : communications in free radical research* vol. 26,1 (2021): 184-189. doi:10.1080/13510002.2021.1999126

[370] Fung, June L et al. "Association of vitamin D intake and serum levels with fertility: results from the Lifestyle and Fertility Study." Fertility and sterility vol. 108,2 (2017): 302-311. doi:10.1016/j.fertnstert.2017.05.037

[371] Ota, Kuniaki et al. "Vitamin D deficiency may be a risk factor for recurrent pregnancy losses by increasing cellular immunity and autoimmunity." Human reproduction (Oxford, England) vol. 29,2 (2014): 208-19. doi:10.1093/humrep/det424

[372] Rudick, Briana J et al. "Influence of vitamin D levels on in vitro fertilization outcomes in donor-recipient cycles." Fertility and sterility vol. 101,2 (2014): 447-52. doi:10.1016/j.fertnstert.2013.10.008

[373] Ota, Kuniaki et al. "Vitamin D deficiency may be a risk factor for recurrent pregnancy losses by increasing cellular immunity and autoimmunity." Human reproduction (Oxford, England) vol. 29,2 (2014): 208-19. doi:10.1093/humrep/det424

[374] Lerchbaum, Elisabeth, and Barbara Obermayer-Pietsch. "Vitamin D and fertility: a systematic review." European journal of endocrinology vol. 166,5 (2012): 765-78. doi:10.1530/EJE-11-0984

[375] Merhi, Zaher O et al. "Circulating vitamin D correlates with serum antimüllerian hormone levels in late-reproductive-aged women: Women's Interagency HIV Study." Fertility and sterility vol. 98,1 (2012): 228-34. doi:10.1016/j.fertnstert.2012.03.029

[376] Drakopoulos, Panagiotis et al. "The effect of serum vitamin D levels on ovarian reserve markers: a prospective cross-sectional study." Human reproduction (Oxford, England) vol. 32,1 (2017): 208-214. doi:10.1093/humrep/dew304

[377] Koga, Fumitoshi et al. "Relationship between nutrition and reproduction." Reproductive medicine and biology vol. 19,3 254-264. 15 Jun. 2020, doi:10.1002/rmb2.12332

[378] van de Vijver, Arne et al. "Vitamin D deficiency and pregnancy rates following frozen-thawed embryo transfer: a prospective cohort study." Human reproduction (Oxford, England) vol. 31,8 (2016): 1749-54. doi:10.1093/humrep/dew107

[379] Franasiak, Jason M et al. "Vitamin D levels do not affect IVF outcomes following the transfer of euploid blastocysts." American journal of obstetrics and gynecology vol. 212,3 (2015): 315.e1-6. doi:10.1016/j.ajog.2014.09.029

[380] Chu, Justin et al. "Vitamin D and assisted reproductive treatment outcome: a systematic review and meta-analysis." Human reproduction (Oxford, England) vol. 33,1 (2018): 65-80. doi:10.1093/humrep/dex326

[381] de Angelis, Cristina et al. "The role of vitamin D in male fertility: A focus on the testis." Reviews in endocrine & metabolic disorders vol. 18,3 (2017): 285-305. doi:10.1007/s11154-017-9425-0

[382] Lerchbaum, Elisabeth, and Barbara Obermayer-Pietsch. "Vitamin D and fertility: a systematic review." European journal of endocrinology vol. 166,5 (2012): 765-78. doi:10.1530/EJE-11-0984

[383] Cito, Gianmartin et al. "Vitamin D and Male Fertility: An Updated Review." The world journal of men's health vol. 38,2 (2020): 164-177. doi:10.5534/wjmh.190057

[384] https://ods.od.nih.gov/HealthInformation/Dietary_Reference_Intakes.aspx

[385] https://ods.od.nih.gov/factsheets/VitaminD/

[386] Cicek, Nedim et al. "Vitamin E effect on controlled ovarian stimulation of unexplained infertile women." Journal of assisted reproduction and genetics vol. 29,4 (2012): 325-8. doi:10.1007/s10815-012-9714-1

[387] Suleiman, S A et al. "Lipid peroxidation and human sperm motility: protective role of vitamin E." Journal of andrology vol. 17,5 (1996): 530-7.

[388] Kessopoulou, E et al. "A double-blind randomized placebo cross-over controlled trial using the antioxidant vitamin E to treat reactive oxygen species associated male infertility." Fertility and sterility vol. 64,4 (1995): 825-31. doi:10.1016/s0015-0282(16)57861-3

[389] Sadaghiani, Safa et al. "Effect of antioxidant supplements on sperm parameters in infertile male smokers: a single-blinded clinical trial." AIMS public health vol. 7,1 92-99. 11 Feb. 2020, doi:10.3934/publichealth.2020009

[390] Moslemi, Mohammad K, and Samaneh Tavanbakhsh. "Selenium-vitamin E supplementation in infertile men: effects on semen parameters and pregnancy rate." International journal of general medicine vol. 4 99-104. 23 Jan. 2011, doi:10.2147/IJGM.S16275

[391] https://ods.od.nih.gov/factsheets/VitaminE-HealthProfessional/

[392] Taş, Sibel et al. "Vitamin B6 supplementation improves oxidative stress and enhances serum paraoxonase/arylesterase activities in streptozotocin-induced diabetic rats." *TheScientificWorldJournal* vol. 2014 (2014): 351598. doi:10.1155/2014/351598

[393] Grajecki, Donata et al. "The effect of micronutrient supplements on female fertility: a systematic review." Archives of gynecology and obstetrics vol. 285,5 (2012): 1463-71. doi:10.1007/s00404-012-2237-2

[394] https://ods.od.nih.gov/factsheets/VitaminB6-HealthProfessional/

[395] https://www.cdc.gov/ncbddd/folicacid/features/folic-acid-helps-prevent-some-birth-defects.html#:~:text=CDC%20urges%20all%20women%20of,are%20anencephaly%20and%20spina%20bifida.

[396] La Vecchia, Irene et al. "Folate, homocysteine and selected vitamins and minerals status in infertile women." The European journal of contraception & reproductive health care : the official journal of the European Society of Contraception vol. 22,1 (2017): 70-75. doi:10.1080/13625187.2016.1263292

[397] Cueto, H T et al. "Folic acid supplementation and fecundability: a Danish prospective cohort study." European journal of clinical nutrition vol. 70,1 (2016): 66-71. doi:10.1038/ejcn.2015.94

[398] Gaskins, Audrey J et al. "Maternal prepregnancy folate intake and risk of spontaneous abortion and stillbirth." Obstetrics and gynecology vol. 124,1 (2014): 23-31. doi:10.1097/AOG.0000000000000343

[399] Balogun, Olukunmi O et al. "Vitamin supplementation for preventing miscarriage." The Cochrane database of systematic reviews vol. 2016,5 CD004073. 6 May. 2016, doi:10.1002/14651858.CD004073.pub4

[400] Gaskins, Audrey J et al. "Dietary folate and reproductive success among women undergoing assisted reproduction." Obstetrics and gynecology vol. 124,4 (2014): 801-809. doi:10.1097/AOG.0000000000000477

---

[401] Kadir, Mumta et al. "Folate intake and ovarian reserve among women attending a fertility center." *Fertility and sterility* vol. 117,1 (2022): 171-180. doi:10.1016/j.fertnstert.2021.09.037

[402] Ebisch, I M W et al. "The importance of folate, zinc and antioxidants in the pathogenesis and prevention of subfertility." Human reproduction update vol. 13,2 (2007): 163-74. doi:10.1093/humupd/dml054

[403] Boxmeer, Jolanda C et al. "Low folate in seminal plasma is associated with increased sperm DNA damage." Fertility and sterility vol. 92,2 (2009): 548-56. doi:10.1016/j.fertnstert.2008.06.010

[404] Mathieu d'Argent, Emmanuelle et al. "High-Dose Supplementation of Folic Acid in Infertile Men Improves IVF-ICSI Outcomes: A Randomized Controlled Trial (FOLFIV Trial)." Journal of clinical medicine vol. 10,9 1876. 26 Apr. 2021, doi:10.3390/jcm10091876

[405] https://ods.od.nih.gov/factsheets/Folate-HealthProfessional/

[406] van de Lagemaat, Erik E et al. "Vitamin B_{12} in Relation to Oxidative Stress: A Systematic Review." *Nutrients* vol. 11,2 482. 25 Feb. 2019, doi:10.3390/nu11020482

[407] La Vecchia, Irene et al. "Folate, homocysteine and selected vitamins and minerals status in infertile women." The European journal of contraception & reproductive health care : the official journal of the European Society of Contraception vol. 22,1 (2017): 70-75. doi:10.1080/13625187.2016.1263292

[408] Bennett, M. "Vitamin B12 deficiency, infertility and recurrent fetal loss." The Journal of reproductive medicine vol. 46,3 (2001): 209-12.

[409] Banihani, Saleem Ali. "Vitamin B_{12} and Semen Quality." *Biomolecules* vol. 7,2 42. 9 Jun. 2017, doi:10.3390/biom7020042

[410] Beltrame, Flávia Luciana et al. "Vitamin B_{12} Prevents Cimetidine-Induced Androgenic Failure and Damage to Sperm Quality in Rats." *Frontiers in endocrinology* vol. 10 309. 10 Jul. 2019, doi:10.3389/fendo.2019.00309

[411] https://ods.od.nih.gov/factsheets/VitaminB12-HealthProfessional/

[412] Jamilian, Mehri et al. "The Effects of Chromium Supplementation on Endocrine Profiles, Biomarkers of Inflammation, and Oxidative Stress in Women with Polycystic Ovary Syndrome: a Randomized, Double-Blind, Placebo-Controlled Trial." *Biological trace element research* vol. 172,1 (2016): 72-78. doi:10.1007/s12011-015-0570-6

[413] Amiri Siavashani, Mehrnush et al. "The Effects of Chromium Supplementation on Gene Expression of Insulin, Lipid, and Inflammatory Markers in Infertile Women With Polycystic Ovary Syndrome Candidate for *in vitro* Fertilization: A Randomized, Double-Blinded, Placebo-Controlled Trial." *Frontiers in endocrinology* vol. 9 726. 28 Nov. 2018, doi:10.3389/fendo.2018.00726

[414] https://ods.od.nih.gov/factsheets/Chromium-HealthProfessional/

[415] Ebisch, I M W et al. "The importance of folate, zinc and antioxidants in the pathogenesis and prevention of subfertility." Human reproduction update vol. 13,2 (2007): 163-74. doi:10.1093/humupd/dml054

[416] Grieger, Jessica A et al. "Maternal Selenium, Copper and Zinc Concentrations in Early Pregnancy, and the Association with Fertility." Nutrients vol. 11,7 1609. 16 Jul. 2019, doi:10.3390/nu11071609

[417] Mori, Rintaro et al. "Zinc supplementation for improving pregnancy and infant outcome." The Cochrane database of systematic reviews ,7 CD000230. 11 Jul. 2012, doi:10.1002/14651858.CD000230.pub4

[418] Ebisch, I M W et al. "The importance of folate, zinc and antioxidants in the pathogenesis and prevention of subfertility." Human reproduction update vol. 13,2 (2007): 163-74. doi:10.1093/humupd/dml054

[419] Fallah, Ali et al. "Zinc is an Essential Element for Male Fertility: A Review of Zn Roles in Men's Health, Germination, Sperm Quality, and Fertilization." Journal of reproduction & infertility vol. 19,2 (2018): 69-81.

[420] Zhao, Jiang et al. "Zinc levels in seminal plasma and their correlation with male infertility: A systematic review and meta-analysis." Scientific reports vol. 6 22386. 2 Mar. 2016, doi:10.1038/srep22386

[421] Yuyan, Li et al. "Are serum zinc and copper levels related to semen quality?." Fertility and sterility vol. 89,4 (2008): 1008-11. doi:10.1016/j.fertnstert.2007.04.028

[422] Omu, A E et al. "Treatment of asthenozoospermia with zinc sulphate: andrological, immunological and obstetric outcome." European journal of obstetrics, gynecology, and reproductive biology vol. 79,2 (1998): 179-84. doi:10.1016/s0301-2115(97)00262-5

[423] Wong, Wai Yee et al. "Effects of folic acid and zinc sulfate on male factor subfertility: a double-blind, randomized, placebo-controlled trial." Fertility and sterility vol. 77,3 (2002): 491-8. doi:10.1016/s0015-0282(01)03229-0

[424] Ebisch, I M W et al. "Does folic acid and zinc sulphate intervention affect endocrine parameters and sperm characteristics in men?." International journal of andrology vol. 29,2 (2006): 339-45. doi:10.1111/j.1365-2605.2005.00598.x

[425] Irani, Morvarid et al. "The Effect of Folate and Folate Plus Zinc Supplementation on Endocrine Parameters and Sperm Characteristics in Sub-Fertile Men: A Systematic Review and Meta-Analysis." Urology journal vol. 14,5 4069-4078. 29 Aug. 2017

[426] Schisterman, Enrique F et al. "Effect of Folic Acid and Zinc Supplementation in Men on Semen Quality and Live Birth Among Couples Undergoing Infertility Treatment: A Randomized Clinical Trial." JAMA vol. 323,1 (2020): 35-48. doi:10.1001/jama.2019.18714

[427] Torres-Arce, Elizabeth et al. "Dietary Antioxidants in the Treatment of Male Infertility: Counteracting Oxidative Stress." Biology vol. 10,3 241. 20 Mar. 2021, doi:10.3390/biology10030241

[428] https://ods.od.nih.gov/factsheets/Zinc-HealthProfessional/

[429] Grieger, Jessica A et al. "Maternal Selenium, Copper and Zinc Concentrations in Early Pregnancy, and the Association with Fertility." Nutrients vol. 11,7 1609. 16 Jul. 2019, doi:10.3390/nu11071609

[430] Qazi, Izhar Hyder et al. "Selenium, Selenoproteins, and Female Reproduction: A Review." Molecules (Basel, Switzerland) vol. 23,12 3053. 22 Nov. 2018, doi:10.3390/molecules23123053

[431] Rayman, Margaret P et al. "Effect of long-term selenium supplementation on mortality: Results from a multiple-dose, randomised controlled trial." Free radical biology & medicine vol. 127 (2018): 46-54. doi:10.1016/j.freeradbiomed.2018.02.015

[432] Torres-Arce, Elizabeth et al. "Dietary Antioxidants in the Treatment of Male Infertility: Counteracting Oxidative Stress." Biology vol. 10,3 241. 20 Mar. 2021, doi:10.3390/biology10030241

[433] Scott, R et al. "The effect of oral selenium supplementation on human sperm motility." British journal of urology vol. 82,1 (1998): 76-80. doi:10.1046/j.1464-410x.1998.00683.x

[434] Safarinejad, Mohammad Reza, and Shiva Safarinejad. "Efficacy of selenium and/or N-acetyl-cysteine for improving semen parameters in infertile men: a

double-blind, placebo controlled, randomized study." The Journal of urology vol. 181,2 (2009): 741-51. doi:10.1016/j.juro.2008.10.015

[435] Cannarella, Rossella et al. "Effects of Selenium Supplementation on Sperm Parameters and DNA-Fragmentation Rate in Patients with Chronic Autoimmune Thyroiditis." Journal of clinical medicine vol. 10,16 3755. 23 Aug. 2021, doi:10.3390/jcm10163755

[436] Bleau, G et al. "Semen selenium and human fertility." Fertility and sterility vol. 42,6 (1984): 890-4.

[437] Hawkes, Wayne Chris et al. "Selenium supplementation does not affect testicular selenium status or semen quality in North American men." Journal of andrology vol. 30,5 (2009): 525-33. doi:10.2164/jandrol.108.006940

[438] https://ods.od.nih.gov/factsheets/Selenium-HealthProfessional/

[439] Tiseo, Bruno C et al. "Coenzyme Q10 Intake From Food and Semen Parameters in a Subfertile Population." *Urology* vol. 102 (2017): 100-105. doi:10.1016/j.urology.2016.11.022

[440] Florou, Panagiota et al. "Does coenzyme Q10 supplementation improve fertility outcomes in women undergoing assisted reproductive technology procedures? A systematic review and meta-analysis of randomized-controlled trials." Journal of assisted reproduction and genetics vol. 37,10 (2020): 2377-2387. doi:10.1007/s10815-020-01906-3

[441] Budani, Maria Cristina, and Gian Mario Tiboni. "Effects of Supplementation with Natural Antioxidants on Oocytes and Preimplantation Embryos." Antioxidants (Basel, Switzerland) vol. 9,7 612. 12 Jul. 2020, doi:10.3390/antiox9070612

[442] Tiseo, Bruno C et al. "Coenzyme Q10 Intake From Food and Semen Parameters in a Subfertile Population." Urology vol. 102 (2017): 100-105. doi:10.1016/j.urology.2016.11.022

[443] Balercia, G et al. "Coenzyme Q10 and male infertility." Journal of endocrinological investigation vol. 32,7 (2009): 626-32. doi:10.1007/BF03346521

[444] Gvozdjáková, Anna et al. "Coenzyme Q_{10}, α-tocopherol, and oxidative stress could be important metabolic biomarkers of male infertility." Disease markers vol. 2015 (2015): 827941. doi:10.1155/2015/827941

[445] Lafuente, Rafael et al. "Coenzyme Q10 and male infertility: a meta-analysis." Journal of assisted reproduction and genetics vol. 30,9 (2013): 1147-56. doi:10.1007/s10815-013-0047-5

[446] Tiseo, Bruno C et al. "Coenzyme Q10 Intake From Food and Semen Parameters in a Subfertile Population." Urology vol. 102 (2017): 100-105. doi:10.1016/j.urology.2016.11.022

[447] https://www.nccih.nih.gov/health/coenzyme-q10

[448] Keller, U et al. "Carnitine status of pregnant women: effect of carnitine supplementation and correlation between iron status and plasma carnitine concentration." *European journal of clinical nutrition* vol. 63,9 (2009): 1098-105. doi:10.1038/ejcn.2009.36

[449] Ku, Chee Wai et al. "Spontaneous miscarriage in first trimester pregnancy is associated with altered urinary metabolite profile." *BBA clinical* vol. 8 48-55. 19 Aug. 2017, doi:10.1016/j.bbacli.2017.07.003

[450] De Luca, Maria Nunzia et al. "Oxidative Stress and Male Fertility: Role of Antioxidants and Inositols." Antioxidants (Basel, Switzerland) vol. 10,8 1283. 13 Aug. 2021, doi:10.3390/antiox10081283

[451] Zhou, Xin et al. "Effect of L-carnitine and/or L-acetyl-carnitine in nutrition treatment for male infertility: a systematic review." Asia Pacific journal of clinical nutrition vol. 16 Suppl 1 (2007): 383-90.

[452] Koeth, Robert A et al. "l-Carnitine in omnivorous diets induces an atherogenic gut microbial pathway in humans." *The Journal of clinical investigation* vol. 129,1 (2019): 373-387. doi:10.1172/JCI94601

[453] https://ods.od.nih.gov/factsheets/Carnitine-HealthProfessional/

[454] Claustrat, B, and J Leston. "Melatonin: Physiological effects in humans." Neuro-Chirurgie vol. 61,2-3 (2015): 77-84. doi:10.1016/j.neuchi.2015.03.002

[455] Hu, Kai-Lun et al. "Melatonin Application in Assisted Reproductive Technology: A Systematic Review and Meta-Analysis of Randomized Trials." Frontiers in endocrinology vol. 11 160. 27 Mar. 2020, doi:10.3389/fendo.2020.00160

[456] Awad, Hosni et al. "Melatonin hormone profile in infertile males." International journal of andrology vol. 29,3 (2006): 409-13. doi:10.1111/j.1365-2605.2005.00624.x

[457] Malmir, Mahdi et al. "Ameliorative effect of melatonin on apoptosis, DNA fragmentation, membrane integrity and lipid peroxidation of spermatozoa in the idiopathic asthenoteratospermic men: In vitro." Andrologia vol. 53,2 (2021): e13944. doi:10.1111/and.13944

[458] H Hassan, Mohammed et al. "Men with idiopathic oligoasthenoteratozoospermia exhibit lower serum and seminal plasma melatonin levels: Comparative effect of night-light exposure with fertile males." Experimental and therapeutic medicine vol. 20,1 (2020): 235-242. doi:10.3892/etm.2020.8678

[459] Meng, Xiao et al. "Dietary Sources and Bioactivities of Melatonin." Nutrients vol. 9,4 367. 7 Apr. 2017, doi:10.3390/nu9040367

[460] https://www.nccih.nih.gov/health/melatonin-what-you-need-to-know

[461] De Luca, Maria Nunzia et al. "Oxidative Stress and Male Fertility: Role of Antioxidants and Inositols." Antioxidants (Basel, Switzerland) vol. 10,8 1283. 13 Aug. 2021, doi:10.3390/antiox10081283

[462] Russo, Michele et al. "Melatonin and Myo-Inositol: Supporting Reproduction from the Oocyte to Birth." *International journal of molecular sciences* vol. 22,16 8433. 5 Aug. 2021, doi:10.3390/ijms22168433

[463] Sortino, Maria A et al. "Polycystic Ovary Syndrome: Insights into the Therapeutic Approach with Inositols." Frontiers in pharmacology vol. 8 341. 8 Jun. 2017, doi:10.3389/fphar.2017.00341

[464] Merviel, Philippe et al. "Impact of myo-inositol treatment in women with polycystic ovary syndrome in assisted reproductive technologies." Reproductive health vol. 18,1 13. 19 Jan. 2021, doi:10.1186/s12978-021-01073-3

[465] Zheng, Xiangqin et al. "Inositol supplement improves clinical pregnancy rate in infertile women undergoing ovulation induction for ICSI or IVF-ET." Medicine vol. 96,49 (2017): e8842. doi:10.1097/MD.0000000000008842

[466] Russo, Michele et al. "Melatonin and Myo-Inositol: Supporting Reproduction from the Oocyte to Birth." International journal of molecular sciences vol. 22,16 8433. 5 Aug. 2021, doi:10.3390/ijms22168433

[467] De Luca, Maria Nunzia et al. "Oxidative Stress and Male Fertility: Role of Antioxidants and Inositols." Antioxidants (Basel, Switzerland) vol. 10,8 1283. 13 Aug. 2021, doi:10.3390/antiox10081283

[468] De Luca, Maria Nunzia et al. "Oxidative Stress and Male Fertility: Role of Antioxidants and Inositols." Antioxidants (Basel, Switzerland) vol. 10,8 1283. 13 Aug. 2021, doi:10.3390/antiox10081283

[469] Formoso, Gloria et al. "Inositol and antioxidant supplementation: Safety and efficacy in pregnancy." Diabetes/metabolism research and reviews vol. 35,5 (2019): e3154. doi:10.1002/dmrr.3154

[470] Carlomagno, G, and V Unfer. "Inositol safety: clinical evidences." European review for medical and pharmacological sciences vol. 15,8 (2011): 931-6.

[471] Formoso, Gloria et al. "Inositol and antioxidant supplementation: Safety and efficacy in pregnancy." Diabetes/metabolism research and reviews vol. 35,5 (2019): e3154. doi:10.1002/dmrr.3154

[472] Takasaki, Akihisa et al. "Endometrial growth and uterine blood flow: a pilot study for improving endometrial thickness in the patients with a thin endometrium." *Fertility and sterility* vol. 93,6 (2010): 1851-8. doi:10.1016/j.fertnstert.2008.12.062

[473] Monari, Francesca et al. "Effect of L-Arginine supplementation in pregnant women with chronic hypertension and previous placenta vascular disorders receiving Aspirin prophylaxis: a randomized control trial." *Minerva obstetrics and gynecology*, 10.23736/S2724-606X.21.04827-2. 12 May. 2021, doi:10.23736/S2724-606X.21.04827-2

[474] Srivastava, Sudha et al. "Mechanism of action of L-arginine on the vitality of spermatozoa is primarily through increased biosynthesis of nitric oxide." Biology of reproduction vol. 74,5 (2006): 954-8. doi:10.1095/biolreprod.105.046896

[475] De Luca, Maria Nunzia et al. "Oxidative Stress and Male Fertility: Role of Antioxidants and Inositols." Antioxidants (Basel, Switzerland) vol. 10,8 1283. 13 Aug. 2021, doi:10.3390/antiox10081283

[476] https://ods.od.nih.gov/factsheets/ExerciseAndAthleticPerformance-HealthProfessional/

[477] https://www.fda.gov/food/cfsan-constituent-updates/fda-sends-warning-letters-seven-companies-illegally-selling-hangover-products

[478] Amin, Ahmed F et al. "N-acetyl cysteine for treatment of recurrent unexplained pregnancy loss." *Reproductive biomedicine online* vol. 17,5 (2008): 722-6. doi:10.1016/s1472-6483(10)60322-7

[479] Badawy, Ahmed et al. "N-Acetyl cysteine and clomiphene citrate for induction of ovulation in polycystic ovary syndrome: a cross-over trial." *Acta obstetricia et gynecologica Scandinavica* vol. 86,2 (2007): 218-22. doi:10.1080/00016340601090337

[480] De Luca, Maria Nunzia et al. "Oxidative Stress and Male Fertility: Role of Antioxidants and Inositols." Antioxidants (Basel, Switzerland) vol. 10,8 1283. 13 Aug. 2021, doi:10.3390/antiox10081283

[481] https://ods.od.nih.gov/factsheets/COVID19-HealthProfessional/#h8

[482] Liu, Mengyuan et al. "Resveratrol protects against age-associated infertility in mice." *Human reproduction (Oxford, England)* vol. 28,3 (2013): 707-17. doi:10.1093/humrep/des437

[483] Ortega, Israel, and Antoni J Duleba. "Ovarian actions of resveratrol." *Annals of the New York Academy of Sciences* vol. 1348,1 (2015): 86-96. doi:10.1111/nyas.12875

[484] Salehi, Bahare et al. "Resveratrol: A Double-Edged Sword in Health Benefits." Biomedicines vol. 6,3 91. 9 Sep. 2018, doi:10.3390/biomedicines6030091

[485] Ochiai, Asako, and Keiji Kuroda. "Preconception resveratrol intake against infertility: Friend or foe?." *Reproductive medicine and biology* vol. 19,2 107-113. 12 Oct. 2019, doi:10.1002/rmb2.12303

[486] Moreira-Pinto, Beatriz et al. "Low Doses of Resveratrol Protect Human Granulosa Cells from Induced-Oxidative Stress." *Antioxidants (Basel, Switzerland)* vol. 10,4 561. 4 Apr. 2021, doi:10.3390/antiox10040561

[487] Ochiai, Asako, and Keiji Kuroda. "Preconception resveratrol intake against infertility: Friend or foe?." *Reproductive medicine and biology* vol. 19,2 107-113. 12 Oct. 2019, doi:10.1002/rmb2.12303

[488] Banaszewska, Beata et al. "Effects of Resveratrol on Polycystic Ovary Syndrome: A Double-blind, Randomized, Placebo-controlled Trial." *The Journal of clinical endocrinology and metabolism* vol. 101,11 (2016): 4322-4328. doi:10.1210/jc.2016-1858

[489] Dull, Ana-Maria et al. "Therapeutic Approaches of Resveratrol on Endometriosis via Anti-Inflammatory and Anti-Angiogenic Pathways." Molecules (Basel, Switzerland) vol. 24,4 667. 13 Feb. 2019, doi:10.3390/molecules24040667

[490]Ochiai, Asako, and Keiji Kuroda. "Preconception resveratrol intake against infertility: Friend or foe?." *Reproductive medicine and biology* vol. 19,2 107-113. 12 Oct. 2019, doi:10.1002/rmb2.12303

[491] Ochiai, Asako et al. "Influence of resveratrol supplementation on IVF-embryo transfer cycle outcomes." *Reproductive biomedicine online* vol. 39,2 (2019): 205-210. doi:10.1016/j.rbmo.2019.03.205

[492] Mestre Citrinovitz, Ana Cecilia et al. "Resveratrol enhances decidualization of human endometrial stromal cells." *Reproduction (Cambridge, England)* vol. 159,4 (2020): 453-463. doi:10.1530/REP-19-0425

[493] Kuroda, Keiji et al. "The actions of resveratrol in decidualizing endometrium: acceleration or inhibition?†." *Biology of reproduction* vol. 103,6 (2020): 1152-1156. doi:10.1093/biolre/ioaa172

[494] Ochiai, Asako, and Keiji Kuroda. "Preconception resveratrol intake against infertility: Friend or foe?." *Reproductive medicine and biology* vol. 19,2 107-113. 12 Oct. 2019, doi:10.1002/rmb2.12303

[495] Garcez, Marcia E et al. "Effects of resveratrol supplementation on cryopreservation medium of human semen." Fertility and sterility vol. 94,6 (2010): 2118-21. doi:10.1016/j.fertnstert.2010.01.058

[496] Archana, D et al. "Alleviative effect of resveratrol on polyvinyl chloride-induced reproductive toxicity in male Wistar rats." Food and chemical toxicology : an international journal published for the British Industrial Biological Research Association vol. 116,Pt B (2018): 173-181. doi:10.1016/j.fct.2018.04.026

[497] Katen, Aimee L et al. "Chronic acrylamide exposure in male mice induces DNA damage to spermatozoa; Potential for amelioration by resveratrol." Reproductive toxicology (Elmsford, N.Y.) vol. 63 (2016): 1-12. doi:10.1016/j.reprotox.2016.05.004

[498] Ourique, Giovana M et al. "Resveratrol prevents oxidative damage and loss of sperm motility induced by long-term treatment with valproic acid in Wistar rats." Experimental and toxicologic pathology : official journal of the Gesellschaft fur Toxikologische Pathologie vol. 68,8 (2016): 435-43. doi:10.1016/j.etp.2016.07.001

[499] Simas, Joana N et al. "Resveratrol improves sperm DNA quality and reproductive capacity in type 1 diabetes." Andrology vol. 9,1 (2021): 384-399. doi:10.1111/andr.12891

[500] https://lpi.oregonstate.edu/mic/dietary-factors/phytochemicals/resveratrol

[501] https://medlineplus.gov/druginfo/natural/307.html

[502] Di Tucci, Chiara et al. "The role of alpha lipoic acid in female and male infertility: a systematic review." Gynecological endocrinology : the official journal of the International Society of Gynecological Endocrinology vol. 37,6 (2021): 497-505. doi:10.1080/09513590.2020.1843619

[503] Haghighian, Hossein Khadem et al. "Randomized, triple-blind, placebo-controlled clinical trial examining the effects of alpha-lipoic acid supplement on the spermatogram and seminal oxidative stress in infertile men." Fertility and sterility vol. 104,2 (2015): 318-24. doi:10.1016/j.fertnstert.2015.05.014

[504] Asa, Elham et al. "Supplementation of freezing media with alpha lipoic acid preserves the structural and functional characteristics of sperm against cryodamage in infertile men with asthenoteratozoospermia." Cryobiology vol. 96 (2020): 166-174. doi:10.1016/j.cryobiol.2020.07.001

[505] Taherian, Samira-Sadat et al. "Alpha-lipoic acid minimises reactive oxygen species-induced damages during sperm processing." Andrologia vol. 51,8 (2019): e13314. doi:10.1111/and.13314

[506] Rago, R et al. "Controlled, prospective, observational study on the efficiency and tolerability of a combination of potential Nrf2-inducing antioxidants and micronutrients as pre-treatment for ICSI in dyspermic patients with previous failure." European review for medical and pharmacological sciences vol. 21,7 (2017): 1645-1652.

[507] Parente, E et al. "Safety of oral alpha-lipoic acid treatment in pregnant women: a retrospective observational study." European review for medical and pharmacological sciences vol. 21,18 (2017): 4219-4227.

[508] https://www.ncbi.nlm.nih.gov/books/NBK564301/

[509] Gharagozloo, Parviz, and R John Aitken. "The role of sperm oxidative stress in male infertility and the significance of oral antioxidant therapy." Human reproduction (Oxford, England) vol. 26,7 (2011): 1628-40. doi:10.1093/humrep/der132

[510] Majzoub, Ahmad, and Ashok Agarwal. "Systematic review of antioxidant types and doses in male infertility: Benefits on semen parameters, advanced sperm function, assisted reproduction and live-birth rate." Arab journal of urology vol. 16,1 113-124. 2 Jan. 2018, doi:10.1016/j.aju.2017.11.013

[511] Nassan, Feiby L et al. "Diet and men's fertility: does diet affect sperm quality?." Fertility and sterility vol. 110,4 (2018): 570-577. doi:10.1016/j.fertnstert.2018.05.025

[512] Agarwal, Ashok et al. "Utility of Antioxidants in the Treatment of Male Infertility: Clinical Guidelines Based on a Systematic Review and Analysis of Evidence." The world journal of men's health vol. 39,2 (2021): 233-290. doi:10.5534/wjmh.200196

[513] Scaruffi, Paola et al. "Oral Antioxidant Treatment of Men Significantly Improves the Reproductive Outcome of IVF Cycles." *Journal of clinical medicine* vol. 10,15 3254. 23 Jul. 2021, doi:10.3390/jcm10153254

[514] Schaefer, Ella, and Deborah Nock. "The Impact of Preconceptional Multiple-Micronutrient Supplementation on Female Fertility." Clinical medicine insights. Women's health vol. 12 1179562X19843868. 23 Apr. 2019, doi:10.1177/1179562X19843868

[515] Agarwal, Ashok et al. "Utility of Antioxidants in the Treatment of Male Infertility: Clinical Guidelines Based on a Systematic Review and Analysis of Evidence." The world journal of men's health vol. 39,2 (2021): 233-290. doi:10.5534/wjmh.200196

[516] Sadaghiani, Safa et al. "Effect of antioxidant supplements on sperm parameters in infertile male smokers: a single-blinded clinical trial." AIMS public health vol. 7,1 92-99. 11 Feb. 2020, doi:10.3934/publichealth.2020009

[517] Russo, Michele et al. "Melatonin and Myo-Inositol: Supporting Reproduction from the Oocyte to Birth." International journal of molecular sciences vol. 22,16 8433. 5 Aug. 2021, doi:10.3390/ijms22168433

[518] Palafox-Carlos, Hugo et al. "The role of dietary fiber in the bioaccessibility and bioavailability of fruit and vegetable antioxidants." *Journal of food science* vol. 76,1 (2011): R6-R15. doi:10.1111/j.1750-3841.2010.01957.x

[519] https://www.dietaryguidelines.gov/

[520] https://www.myplate.gov/

[521] Erland, Lauren A E, and Praveen K Saxena. "Melatonin Natural Health Products and Supplements: Presence of Serotonin and Significant Variability of Melatonin Content." *Journal of clinical sleep medicine : JCSM : official publication of the American Academy of Sleep Medicine* vol. 13,2 275-281. 15 Feb. 2017, doi:10.5664/jcsm.6462

[522] https://www.consumerreports.org/supplements/how-to-choose-supplements-wisely-a2238386100/

[523] Henkel, Ralf et al. "The excessive use of antioxidant therapy: A possible cause of male infertility?." Andrologia vol. 51,1 (2019): e13162. doi:10.1111/and.13162

[524] Garolla, Andrea et al. "Dietary Supplements for Male Infertility: A Critical Evaluation of Their Composition." Nutrients vol. 12,5 1472. 19 May. 2020, doi:10.3390/nu12051472

[525] https://ods.od.nih.gov/factsheets/list-all/.

[526] Brotman, Rebecca M et al. "The effect of vaginal douching cessation on bacterial vaginosis: a pilot study." American journal of obstetrics and gynecology vol. 198,6 (2008): 628.e1-7. doi:10.1016/j.ajog.2007.11.043

[527] https://www.acog.org/womens-health/faqs/pelvic-inflammatory-disease

[528] https://probioticsnow.com/

[529] https://internationalprobiotics.org/

[530] https://www.amazon.com/Globesity-Things-Didnt-Know-Making/dp/146211296X/ref=sr_1_3?crid=Z5OZSX7RAP4E&keywords=globesity&qid=1638573729&sprefix=globesity%2Caps%2C220&sr=8-3

[531] https://probioticsnow.com/

[532] https://www.dietaryguidelines.gov/

[533] https://www.myplate.gov/

Printed in Great Britain
by Amazon

17734168R00193